Finding the Strength Within

Living With Chronic Fatigue Syndrome (ME:CFS)

Debora K. Toll (Ph.D.)

ISBN: 978-1-7773842-0-3 (paperback)

Cover artist: Haley Toll
Company name: R. Zai Art
Title of the artwork: Resilience
Artist's contact information: instagram.com/r.zai.art/?hl=en

Contents

Figures

Tables

Preface

When I was first diagnosed with myalgic encephalomyelitis/chronic fatigue syndrome (ME/CFS), I had no idea what would lie before me. ME/CFS sounded like a rather benign disorder and one that I would recover from quickly. Little did I know that I would face years of profound fatigue and that this disease would express itself with numerous, varied and endless symptoms. Little did I know that this disease would debilitate my life and challenge me deeply at the physical, cognitive and spiritual levels of my being. Little did I know that this disease would be so grueling and demanding that I would no longer know the person who I once was or what my future might hold for me.

I watched myself go from a very active and high energy person to one who could barely get out of bed, from a once optimistic person to one who could barely see any light at the end of the tunnel and from a fairly understanding person to one who struggled to be civil with others. The struggles with: a) the loss of my former self, the person who I believed I was and the person who I loved being, b) my present self, feeling lost and broken and c) my future self, wondering if my health and my life were as good as they were going to get, were often too much to deal with. I experienced many dark days and nights of the soul as a result of this disease.

In addition to the daily and unending struggles with ME/CFS, like so many other individuals living with a chronic and invisible disease, I felt alone and misunderstood. It was often difficult for individuals in my life to understand this disease and how drastically it was impacting my life. I get it!! After all, how bad can having a disease as seemingly as benign as ME/CFS be? Plus, I looked healthy. I would sometimes hear "Deb, you look good, it can't be that bad" or "Deb, everyone is tired". These words could leave me feeling so misunderstood, judged and added to the burden of having this disease. I recall one encounter with an individual who had also been recently diagnosed with ME/CFS. This individual commented "my loved ones are questioning if I am sick or if it is all in my head. I am so discouraged". Comments such as these are not uncommon for patients to hear from the individuals in their life.

Not being familiar with ME/CFS, like the people in my life, I had no goal posts or road map by which to understand or assess my disease experiences so, I began to turn to books on the subject matter and the more "general" information published on internet sites. It was there that I learned that some individuals were able to recover their health within 6 months of diagnosis, through exercise and healthy eating. This information however, left me bewildered and discouraged as my experiences were so different from those accounts. I could barely move or feed myself, and any amount of activity would force me back into bed unable to move for days at a time. Moreover, I was experiencing many symptoms that were not mentioned on the more reputable internet sites. I was very disheartened and started to question "what was wrong with me"?

Over time, I began to review the ME/CFS research literature and it was there that I found answers to my physical, cognitive and spiritual challenges. The research literature spoke to my many symptoms, reported similar patient experiences to mine and explained how this disease differs in patients by the number, type, severity and duration of their symptoms. Individuals who experience a milder case of the disease may indeed, return to their previous health levels fairly, quickly after disease onset. Individuals who experience a more severe case, however, may never return to their premorbid health levels. It was in the research literature that I also discovered that I was on the more moderate to severe end of the disease spectrum and finally, began to feel less alone in my experiences with this disease. ME/CFS, unlike any previous health or life experience, challenged me to the core of my being. It asked me to dig deep and to find the strength within.

In this book, I invite you to join me as I share my patient experiences with the varied and relentless ME/CFS symptoms and their debilitating effects on my life, from the physical, cognitive and spiritual points of view. I also discuss my journey through the research literature and explain how it helped me develop a better understanding of this complex, multi-system disease and my varied experiences both with it and the different treatment approaches. Finally, I share some of my reflections on living with ME/CFS and how I moved forward with my "new" life.

It is my hope that this book will help the reader appreciate what living with a chronic, invisible and debilitating disease is like most particularly, that of ME/CFS. It is also my desire that in sharing my journey with a more moderate to severe disease experience, that the reader will develop a deeper understanding of this challenging and debilitating disease, its devastating and life changing impacts, and its possible patient outcomes, treatments and prognoses. Ultimately, I hope that this book will be a roadmap, a warm embrace and a source of hope for individuals who struggle with this disease. Please know that you are not alone. Finally, I hope that this book will help family members, employers, colleagues and medical professionals alike, develop an understanding of this often misunderstood, devastating, complex, multi-system disease and the individuals who live and struggle with it.

It should be noted at the outset, that this book is written from the lens of a personal journey and in many respects, is a reflective piece. Moreover, the research literature cited addresses the adult experience and represents my journey through the literature to develop a better understanding of this disease, my experiences with it and the possible outcomes, treatments and prognoses. Some readers may thus, argue that this book is not an objective and dispassionate account of the subject matter. Furthermore, as I am not a medical practitioner, I have not critically analyzed nor interpreted the research findings, I have simply reported them. Finally, over the years, this disease has been referred to in a variety of ways such as chronic fatigue immune dysfunction syndrome (CFIDS), Epstein Barr Virus (EBV), Iceland disease, post viral fatigue syndrome (PVFS) and systemic exertion intolerance disease (SEID). The term myalgic encephalomyelitis/chronic fatigue syndrome (ME/CFS) however, has been used most consistently in North America and is increasingly, being used worldwide [1, 2]. In light of this, the term ME/CFS will be used throughout this book.

Acknowledgements

This book would not have come to fruition without the love, support and encouragement of my family and friends. Thanks to each of you for always being there for me and for being kind, thoughtful and loving souls. A special thank you to my nieces and nephews, and their little ones, for bringing so much love, laughter and light into my life. A very, special thank you to my mom and dad for their unconditional love and teaching me to believe in the goodness of life and its endless possibilities. All of you fill my heart with profound love and joy!

An enormous thank you to my niece, Haley Toll, for the lovely artwork on the book jacket. Haley captured the essence of my journey in artform! Thank you, Haley, for your heartfelt and meaningful work. Doctors L. Kozyra and M. Picard-Lessard, thank you so much for your excellent medical advice and support throughout the years. You were a place of solace for me. Dr. B.A. Turpin, thank you for your valuable commentary and assistance with the book's graphics and to my sister Wendy, thank you for your insightful feedback on my drafts. And to Brodi, my dearest four-legged friend, thank you for your patience, insisting that I got my walks and providing me with supportive kisses all along the way. Finally, to the reader, thank you very much for your support! I hope that this book will help you in your ME/CFS journey and to remember that life, no matter what its challenges, is rich with blessings.

A list of commonly cited acronyms

CBT – Cognitive behavioral therapy
CCC – Canadian Consensus Criteria
CDC – U.S. Centers for Disease and Prevention Control
CFS – Chronic fatigue syndrome
EBV – Epstein Barr Virus
FMS – Fibromyalgia syndrome
GET – Graded exercise therapy
IBS – Irritable bowel syndrome
ICC – International Consensus Criteria
MCS – Multiple chemical sensitivities
ME – Myalgic encephalomyelitis
ME/CFS – Myalgic encephalomyelitis/chronic fatigue syndrome
MUPS – Medically unexplained physical symptoms
NICE – British National Institute for Health and Clinical Excellence
NIH – U.S. National Institute of Health
OI – Orthostatic intolerance
PEM – Post exertional malaise
SEID – Systemic exertion intolerance disease
TMJ – Temporomandibular joint pain

Chapter 1

INTRODUCTION

Life is a succession of moments, to live each one is to succeed
~ Corita Kent

Life is 10% what happens to you and 90% how you react to it
~ Charles R. Swindoll

Before discussing my personal journey with myalgic encephalomyelitis/ chronic fatigue syndrome (ME/CFS), I believe that it is important to provide some context for this book. From my perspective, it is important for the reader to appreciate that ME/CFS is a chronic and invisible disease. As we shall discover, this fact can create a number of issues for patients and "others" (e.g., family members, caregivers and medical personnel) in their life. Further, I believe that it is important to understand how ME/CFS is defined and its substantial impacts at the individual, family, medical, economic and societal levels. Finally, I believe it important for the reader to appreciate a little bit about my character and the context of how my journey with ME/CFS began, as they may be germane to other individuals' disease experiences. This chapter will sequentially, explore these subject matters.

ME/CFS: A chronic and invisible disease
ME/CFS is a chronic disease. As such, by definition, it is a disease that lasts for one or more years, requires ongoing medical attention and can limit the activities of the individual's daily life (https://www.cdc.gov/ chronicdisease/about/index.htm). A chronic disease, also known as a

noncommunicable disease, is a disease that is persistent and generally, slow in progression. While these diseases can be treated, they are usually not cured [1]. An invisible disease, on the other hand, is defined as a "physical, mental or neurological condition that is not visible from the outside, yet can limit or challenge a person's movements, senses, or activities" [2]. Invisible diseases include Crohn's, renal failure, arthritis, diabetes, heart disease, fibromyalgia, sleep disorders, ME/CFS and mental illnesses, among others [2]. Chronic and invisible diseases, while not visible from the outside, can be long lasting, non-curable, life limiting and life changing for the individuals who suffer from them.

ME/CFS itself, is defined as a "devastating, multi-system disease that causes dysfunction of the neurological, immune, endocrine and energy/ metabolism systems" [3]. ME/CFS is associated with numerous, varied, relentless and debilitating symptoms such as an overwhelming and debilitating fatigue, chronic pain, cognitive dysfunction, sleep disorders, immune dysfunction, orthostatic dysfunction and post-exertional fatigue and malaise [4, 5]. ME/CFS is regarded as a complex, debilitating and challenging disease that cannot be explained by any underlying medical condition [4, 5].

The impacts of ME/CFS

The impacts of ME/CFS can be far reaching. This disease touches the lives of patients, their loved ones, caregivers, employers, medical and research communities, and economies at large. Worldwide, an estimated 17 million people are believed to suffer from this disease [6]. Among these are an estimated 1.7-3.38 million Americans [7], 260,000 Britons [8] and 560,000 Canadians [9]. The number of people living with ME/ CFS however, is believed to be considerably higher than these estimates. One estimate suggests that 1% of the adult population experiences ME/ CFS [10] while, another estimate suggests that 84-91% of all ME/CFS cases remain undiagnosed [11]. In other words, fewer than 20% of all ME/CFS patients have been diagnosed [12, 13]. In Canada, ME/CFS is believed to be more prevalent than lung cancer and AIDS [14], and more common than heart disease, cancer, Parkinson's and multiple sclerosis combined [9]. ME/CFS may, therefore, touch the lives of many people who we know and love.

The impacts of ME/CFS on the individual patients themselves can be quite extensive. These impacts can include a loss of their quality of life, independence, productivity, income and employment. They can also include a loss of family, social and medical support, higher medical costs and increased work absences. Moreover, ME/CFS is a disease for which public awareness is lacking [15]. As a result, many patients can further face "others'" misunderstandings, false perceptions and judgements about this disease [1, 16]. These misunderstandings, false perceptions and judgements can often translate into "others" wondering if ME/CFS is all in the patients' head, into medical personnel and caregivers questioning if patients are malingering, and in some cases, into doctors misdiagnosing patients. Finally, they can translate into patients feeling alone and stigmatized, further impacting their health and overall sense of well-being.

The economic impacts of ME/CFS can be far reaching as well. The loss of productivity to the U.S. economy for example, is an estimated $9.1 billion per annum [17]. Moreover, the annual cost burden of the direct costs (e.g., office visits, medical tests, medication) and indirect costs (e.g., loss of income and productivity, welfare costs) are estimated at close to $24 billion [18] while, the annual overall costs to families, caregivers, employers and society at large are an estimated $18 – $51 billion U.S. [15]. In the U.S., the patients' average, annual medical costs are believed to be three to four times higher than those of the general populace [6]. All in all, the economic impacts of ME/CFS are believed to be comparable to those of other chronic illnesses, that extract some of the largest medical and socioeconomic costs [19]. The annual cost burden of ME/CFS to the U.K. economy is also quite substantive, sitting at an estimated 3.3 billion pounds [20] while, the annual loss of productivity to the Canadian economy is an estimated $6.82 billion [21]. Research wise, in 2017, the U.S. expended $14 million on ME/CFS research [22, 23] while, the United Kingdom spent 10.17 million pounds between the 2006-2015 time-period [24]. In 2018, Canada set aside $1.8 million for a joint ME/CFS research project with the U.S. [25, 26] and in 2019, the Canadian Institutes of Health Research allocated $1.4 million to create and develop a national research network to study ME/CFS [27]. While some may argue that the level of ME/CFS research funding is adequate, others argue that the funding, commensurate with ME/CFS' disease burden (i.e., number of people affected by an illness and the associated disability and early death rates), is sorely lacking [28], as will be discussed further in Chapter 5. Clearly, the impacts of ME/CFS are extensive, touching the lives of millions of patients, their loved ones, caregivers, employers, medical and research communities, and national economies alike. The impacts of this complex, debilitating and challenging disease ripple throughout many levels of our society.

A little bit about my character and the context of how my journey with ME/CFS began

Character wise, I am a determined, highly motivated and independent person who loves to set and achieve new goals and pursue new adventures. I have long believed that if I could dream a dream, it was achievable. I simply had to believe in my dream, set my intention towards it, work towards it and yes, pray for it. I am also typically, a very positive, high energy and active person. I played all types of sports, was active socially, read and gardened avidly, loved travel, theatre and adventure, was upwardly mobile in my career and continuously strove to be all that I could be, including a more compassionate and kinder soul. I also loved to spend time in nature, taking long walks in the woods and enjoying time on the water. I particularly loved to spend time with my family and friends and found much joy in time spent with my nephews and nieces. Continuous learning was extremely important to me as well. This quest for learning took me to many new life experiences, job opportunities and the completion of my Masters' and Ph.D. degrees. I have long sought to joyfully embrace and fully live my life. Moreover, I believed that I would finish my career as a healthy and vibrant individual, and that my retirement years would be filled with much travel and many new adventures and interests. In 2011 however, two years before my retirement, I was diagnosed with ME/CFS. This disease has subsequently, changed not only my retirement plans but my entire life.

ME/CFS was so life changing that shortly after my ME/CFS diagnosis, I found myself intently examining the years leading up to that diagnosis. I desperately needed to understand if I might have done something to cause this disease or whether there were specific life circumstances that might have triggered it. If so, I needed to understand what they were so that I could address them and quickly recover my health. This examination led to the realization that I had been experiencing numerous health issues prior to my ME/CFS diagnosis. I do not know if these health issues were precursors and led up to my journey with ME/CFS but, I would like to mention them as they may be germane to other peoples' ME/CFS experiences.

For twelve years prior to my ME/CFS diagnosis in 2011, I had been living with another chronic disorder, that of chronic vertigo. Initially, the vertigo was diagnosed as endolymphatic hydrops – a disorder of the vestibular system that, through changes in the volume and composition of the endolymph fluid in the inner ear, causes severe balance problems or vertigo (www.californiaearinstitute.com/ear-disorders-endolymphatic-hydrops). Over time, this diagnosis was changed to chronic vertigo, caused by migraines. The vertigo could, on occasion, be so severe that I would be absent from work for periods of one or two weeks. After a lot of bed rest, the extreme vertigo, nausea, fatigue and migraines would pass, and I could once again, resume my work and life's pleasures. Any overly fatiguing situation, however, could cause a relapse. As a single and financially independent person, I was quite concerned about missing work and was very, fortunate as I had supportive senior managers who allowed me to work from home 1-2 days a week. This work flexibility allowed me to better manage this disorder and along with changes in my personal life (e.g., cutting back on my athletic and social activities) ultimately, reduced my severe vertigo relapses and my time away from the office. I was thus, able to live a fairly, normal life.

The 2005-2011 timeframe was filled with other, physical and emotional challenges as well. During that time, I said goodbye to a number of very dear aunts and uncles, friends and my best friend Cassie, my 14.5, year old cairn terrier. Many of these precious souls had been struggling with their health for years prior to their passing and I tried to be there for them in any way that I could. It was a period of a lot of emotional upheaval and it hurt me deeply to say goodbye to them. I was also facing other health challenges. One of which, was a torn rotator cuff. I lived in a great deal of pain for a couple of years and no amount of massage therapy, physiotherapy or cortisone shots relieved that pain. In 2011, I required surgery to repair my rotator cuff. For the first time in my life, I also had bronchitis and pneumonia, and was struggling with numerous and more severe colds. I began visiting my doctor more frequently, as my immune system was seemingly, becoming more compromised. My energy levels were also starting to wane, and fatigue began to profoundly tax my life. My specialist suggested that the chronic vertigo was likely causing the increased fatigue as my body was having to constantly struggle to remain upright and find its equilibrium. I continued to push through my episodes of vertigo, more frequent illnesses and increasing levels of fatigue, as I did not want to be away from work or diminish my career opportunities. I also wanted to maintain some degree of normalcy in my life, like spending time with my family and friends. Part of my character is to not give up – I could do this – whatever it took! If all else failed, my determination, positive thinking and will-power would carry me through.

As time passed, my energy levels became extremely low and work was increasingly, taking up more and more of my energy and life. All of my evenings, weekends, compensatory time and holidays were now being used to rest and sleep, in order to continue to meet my work demands. Upward mobility was now a thing of my past and time with family, friends and social activities were extremely limited. Moreover, in the last 16 months of my career, work was very demanding. During that time, I was responsible for helping senior managers undertake four reorganizations, over a 14-month period. Each reorganization demanded a high level of physical and cognitive energy on my part. In addition, in the last six months of this project, due to a change in managers, I was no longer able to work from home 1-2 days a week – a key strategy in me maintaining my overall health. Increasingly, I had less and less energy and eventually, work became my first and only choice of energy expenditure. I simply did not have the energy to pursue anything else.

During the three to four months prior to my 2011 summer vacation and my ME/CFS diagnosis, I found myself having less and less energy even for work. It took everything that I had to just get myself to the office. Once there, I just wanted to sit in my chair and do my work. I was too exhausted to take my usual walk at lunch or go and get a cup of tea. It took everything that I had to just get up and go to the washroom or attend a meeting. My adrenaline reserves were very low, if non-existent. I once had abounding energy reserves but now, I wished that I could inject adrenalin into my veins to just get me through my day. By the end of the workday, I had nothing left in me. I started to no longer care to garden, walk my dog Brodi, prepare a meal for myself or even hear from family or friends. I just wanted to be left alone to rest and sleep but, not even rest and sleep were sustaining me any longer. By August 2011, when my summer holidays came due, I could no longer struggle through my fatigue and my energy reserves were non-existent. I was drained! Three days after the start of my summer vacation my body came to an abrupt halt – I could not get out of bed I was so exhausted, weak, nauseated and in pain. And so, my journey with a ME/CFS diagnosis began.

I was unable to return to my workplace and the career that I loved following my summer vacation. I struggled deeply, for the longest time, with my desire to return to work and my inability to do so. Moreover, for almost the first year and a half following my diagnosis, I would frequently hear my inner voice say, "you are such a loser". I finally, began to ask myself why, at some level, do you think that "you are such a loser". The response eluded me for a while and then one day it hit me, "you could not return to your workplace, finish your career or will yourself back to health, back to your life. What is wrong with you?" Wow! At some level, I was angry and disappointed with myself for not being able to change or affect my situation, not even through my usual modus operandi of sheer determination and will power. Furthermore, the struggles with this disease were relentless and so too, was the shame. As hard as I tried, I was physically, cognitively and spiritually incapable of returning to work, to an organization and people that I loved, and I could not explain either to myself or to others why I was so challenged by this disease, what may have caused it, why I was unable to recover my health and what was becoming of me – I was seemingly, so broken, my life so shattered! And the biggest question and perhaps, the greatest shame – did I bring this disease on by not looking after myself sufficiently and if so, how could I have let that happen? I was conscious of the importance of good health and had always tried to live a healthy lifestyle so, what did I miss that lead to this devastating disease? And so, my journey through the ME/CFS research literature began.

As mentioned in the Preface, this book represents an account of my ME/CFS journey from the physical, cognitive and spiritual points of view as well as, my journey through the research literature in search of a deeper understanding of this devastating, complex, multisystem disease and my experiences with it. In Chapter 2, I will share my experiences with the numerous and relentless physical, cognitive and spiritual challenges of this disease and their devastating impacts on my life. In Chapter 3, I will discuss some of the more "general" research literature on what ME/CFS is and how it manifests itself. In this chapter, we will begin to understand some of the complexities of this disease. In Chapter 4, I will share the research findings regarding the core ME/CFS symptom categories and their debilitating effects on patients' lives. In Chapter 4, we will come to understand the challenging, devastating and multi-system aspects of this disease. In Chapter 5, I will discuss some of the other possible patient outcomes and the prognoses of this disease, and in Chapter 6, I will explore some of the treatments that can lead to symptom relief and recovery. Finally, in Chapter 7, I will share some of my reflections on living with this disease and how I was able to move forward with my "new" life.

Chapter 2

MY PHYSICAL, COGNITIVE AND SPIRITUAL CHALLENGES

God gave us the gift of life; it is up to us to give ourselves the gift of living well

~ Voltaire

The spiritual dimension is your center, your commitment to your value system. It draws upon the sources that inspire and uplift you and tie you to timeless truths of humanity

~ Stephen Covey

Life is the immortal flow of energy that nourishes, extends and preserves. Its eternal goal is life

~ Smiley Blanton

Before delving into a discussion of the ME/CFS research literature that helped me to better understand this disease and my experiences with it, I would first like to outline the challenges that I experienced with ME/CFS. I believe that it is important to do so as this was the "natural" progression of my journey with this disease – moving from the experiential to knowledge and understanding.

It has been over nine years since I was diagnosed with ME/CFS and I continue to struggle with this disease. I realize that I am very, fortunate as ME/CFS, unlike so many other diseases, is typically, not life-threatening.

ME/CFS however, can threaten many aspects of an individual's life. In my case, my physical, cognitive and spiritual well-being. ME/CFS has been extremely challenging and life changing for me, and in many respects, it has left my life a small semblance of what it once was. In this chapter, I would like to share some of the physical, cognitive and spiritual challenges that I faced with this chronic, invisible, debilitating and life changing disease.

As mentioned in the Preface, I had no goal posts or road map by which to understand or assess my disease experiences and I was struggling to comprehend why many of the symptoms that I was experiencing were not mentioned on the more reputable internet sites. I was also struggling with why some individuals, through exercise and healthy eating, were reporting a return to their former health levels within six months of disease onset while, I was struggling to just get out of bed for almost the entire first year. I was perplexed and began to question "what was going on with me"? Why were my experiences so different and why was I, unlike the other individuals, unable to overcome this disease and return to the life that I once loved and fully embraced? I was in deep despair and felt lost and broken!

It was only by delving deep into the research literature that I discovered that patients' experiences with ME/CFS can vary substantially, depending on the number, type, severity and duration of their symptoms [1]. Furthermore, the disease spectrum is fairly, broad with some individuals experiencing a mild to moderate case, others a moderate to severe and yet others, a severe to very severe [2]. Depending on the severity of the individuals' disease state, some patients may return to their former health levels fairly, quickly after disease onset while, other patients may struggle for years and yet others, may never return to their premorbid health levels [3]. I also discovered that due to the range and severity of the patients' disease symptoms, their own unique biological needs and their unique responses to treatments, ME/CFS treatment approaches may need to be individualized [4]. All of these research findings, which will be explained in the remaining chapters, helped me to understand that my ME/CFS experiences were on the more moderate to severe end of the disease spectrum, explained my numerous, varied, debilitating and longer lasting symptoms, and helped me to identify the treatment approaches that were most effective for me.

It is my hope that in sharing my ME/CFS journey, the reader will develop a deeper understanding of what a patient experience can entail, most particularly, from the lens of a more moderate to severe disease state. It is also my hope that other individuals will not have to struggle in the manner that I did in trying to understand their many, varied and long lasting symptoms, and why their experiences may be so different from those of other individuals'. This chapter will sequentially address my numerous, varied and more severe physical, cognitive and spiritual challenges with ME/CFS.

My physical challenges

The physical challenges that ME/CFS imposed on my life were numerous, varied, relentless and very debilitating. Of all my physical challenges however, fatigue was by far the most challenging. Over the course of my life, I had experienced other fatiguing disorders such as chronic vertigo, mononucleosis (i.e., Epstein Barr Virus), burn out and depression but, no previous illness experience prepared me for the fatigue levels associated with ME/CFS. In fact, I would never have believed that such levels of fatigue were humanly possible, had I not experienced them myself. I was so profoundly fatigued that I could barely move. For almost the entire first year following my diagnosis, I was, for all intents and purposes, bedridden. I was sleeping 18-20 hours a day! My energy levels were non-existent, and no amount of sleep or rest helped to restore them.

The level of exhaustion in my body was so profound that meeting the simplest of my life's demands was exceedingly, difficult. Preparing something as simple as a tea and toast or a bowl of cereal, was extremely challenging for me. These simple tasks felt insurmountable and only taxed my already depleted energy levels further, leaving me scurrying back to bed for more, endless hours of sleep. Preparing a frozen dinner was no small feat either. There were countless times when I simply could not get back out of bed to take the dinner out of the oven. I found myself wanting to sleep and sleep and sleep a little bit more, before going down the stairs to retrieve my frequently, burned food from the oven. The tiredness was so overwhelming, I could not move or even think of moving. Many times, I recall wishing that my little cairn terrier Brodi, could have cooked for me.

While I know that I could have asked family and friends for help, just the thought of calling them and making the necessary arrangements to drop by, was far too taxing for me. I just needed a lot of sleep, quietude and none of life's demands.

Other, simple daily activities like getting up to go to the washroom, a couple of feet from my bed, was an enormous challenge and so often, was beyond my physical capabilities. It too, was a huge quest that demanded so much of me! Before getting up from bed, I literally, had to lie there and envision energy, ask my body to manifest the energy and when I felt that I had sufficient energy, I would head off down the hallway to the washroom – coaching and telling myself along the way that I could do this. By the time I got back to bed, I was even more exhausted – I just wanted to cry. Other, simple activities like sitting up in a chair to eat a meal, watching television, listening to music and having a short, telephone conversation with a friend were also taxing. I was highly intolerant to any level of physical exertion! A necessary outing, such as a doctor's appointment or a medical test, were particularly challenging and required me to dig deep. I had to push myself extremely hard to get to the office and once there, I had great difficulty functioning. I was so overwhelmed by the fatigue – I could barely move or think. Upon returning home, I faced even more exhaustion and malaise, and was bedridden for days later.

The deep, physical exhaustion permeated everything that I did, making my life one huge struggle. Quite simply, I had no physical stamina and no energy reserves to call upon. Any amount of movement or physical activity was arduous and only served to intensify my fatigue levels further. I, consequently, had to adapt and started to change the way I once did things in my life. I had for example, to hire people to maintain my house and property – things that I once loved to do. Grocery shopping became small, convenience stores, gift shopping became internet shopping, hair appointments, which were now very seldom, became walk-ins and the rest of my life was on hold. So often, I sat in disbelief and despair at how drastically the fatigue was debilitating and devastating my life. My life was now a matter of either not having the energy to do anything, trying to get up sufficient energy to do something or, having to simply wait and see if I might have the necessary energy at a later point in time. Everything in my life was an incredible challenge, requiring me to incessantly, push myself hard and tell myself that I could do this – I felt like I was constantly walking into the headwinds of my life! My bed was my only real place of comfort from the extreme fatigue and the countless, other physical symptoms. In fact, my bed became my sanctuary. I would never have thought that this would be the state of my life, the extent of my physical being. It was surreal! The fatigue of ME/CFS landed me very, hard on my backside both figuratively and literally speaking.

Any physical demand, no matter how seemingly insignificant, exacerbated the extreme fatigue and many of my other physical symptoms. Among these other symptoms was excruciating body pain. As with the fatigue, simple acts like standing up or walking a short distance triggered the extreme pain. At times, the pain in my back was so intense that it literally felt like someone was tearing the muscles away from my bone structure. It was so uncomfortable, debilitating and life limiting. I also experienced incredibly, painful spasms in my legs and neck as well as, terrible cramping and burning in my muscles and joints. A simple touch to my thighs and arms caused so much pain, and I am no wimp when it comes to pain. Moreover, I experienced debilitating pain in my knees and hips particularly when I was using a stairwell or getting into or out of a car. So often, even the soles of my feet and toes hurt and I would, consequently, find myself hobbling around the house in great discomfort. There were many times when even my teeth hurt! Unfortunately, not even sleep was a respite from the pain as a simple leg, arm or neck movement would awaken me. I frequently, needed to get up from bed to take a hot bath and extra strength Tylenol just to get back to sleep but, many nights, not even these approaches relieved the pain and discomfort. Every movement hurt, day and night! It was as though my entire body had a heightened sensitivity to pain and this too, could be exhausting. There was little respite from the profound levels of fatigue and body pain.

In addition to the fatigue and chronic pain, I experienced countless other physical symptoms. Frequent nose bleeds, long-lasting migraines, nausea to the point of dry heaving, dizziness and sleep dysfunction were common occurrences. The sleep dysfunction only added to my already debilitating, fatigue levels. I was either not able to fall asleep for hours on end or I could not remain asleep – I felt like I was waking up every 10 to 15 minutes, throughout the entire night! I also experienced a pressure in my head, trembling in my hands, arms and legs, and overall body weakness. So many times, I felt like my legs would not support me, they were so weak. It was as though there was insufficient oxygen reaching them and countless other times, I could literally feel the oxygen draining from my legs when I stood up or walked. At other times, my legs felt very heavy and moved with difficulty. It was as though I had weights around my ankles. Moreover, when I walked, my leg muscles trembled, I was disoriented, unbalanced and unsure of my footing and frequently, felt like I was going to nose plant into the floor. I also experienced a stiffness in my hands and fingers, dry eyes, blurred vision, earaches, swollen and sore lymph nodes in my neck, irritable bowel, urinary frequency, morning stiffness and a worsening of symptoms with stress. Finally, I experienced labored breathing, panic attacks, heart palpitations and a numbness in my face and left arm.

There were many occasions when I thought that I might be developing a heart problem as my heart frequently, beat faster and the pain in my left chest could be crushing. I recall one night when the pain was so bad, I thought that I was having a heart attack. I distinctly remember being so fatigued and weak that I could not conceive of dialing 911, getting up, getting dressed, getting into the ambulance and heading off to hospital – I was just too exhausted. I recall saying a prayer that I would wake up the next morning and accepted that should I not perhaps, it was just my time. Admittedly, that was not the brightest move on my part but, the level of exhaustion and the physical challenges of getting to hospital overpowered my logic. Admittedly, deep down, I was also counting on the pain in my chest being the result of anxiety, as my recent cardiovascular test results were normal. All this to say, the physical exhaustion and the demands of the other physical symptoms could be so profound that at times, just the thought of movement or activity was inconceivable.

The physical challenges of this disease just kept coming – it was "crazy making". I experienced sensitivities to light, noise and smells as well as, new sensitivities to food and medications. I had extreme intolerances to heat and cold, night chills and sweats, jaw pain, abdominal pain, light headedness, hair loss and color changes in the pigmentation of my skin. Flus were now more severe and required longer recovery periods, and vaccinations left me ill and in bed for sometimes, 7-10 days later. I never knew what to expect next, the physical challenges of this disease were so numerous, ever changing, relentless and debilitating. It was as though my body's alarm panel was all lit up with sirens blaring but, I did not possess the necessary override code. I was so uncomfortable in my own body – it was now foreign to me. I was bewildered, disillusioned and overwrought by the many, physical symptoms that I was experiencing.

At one point in time, I was pretty much up for anything in order to regain some semblance of my former life. In an attempt to do so, I tried to undertake some light exercises, as my primary doctor, my general practitioner (GP), had recommended. I thought, I can do this, as I dragged myself down to my tread mill in the basement. Unfortunately, after 2-3 minutes of light walking on the treadmill, I was pooped. My hands were shaking, my head was aching, my nose was bleeding, I was weak, dizzy and nauseated, and my back and chest were sore. I could barely make it back up the basement stairs to the main floor as my legs were weak, trembling and in pain. I was also huffing and puffing along the way – my breathing was so labored. As I sat at the bottom of the stairs on the main floor, I thought energy, commanded some energy, told myself I could do this and asked God for help. I then continued my quest of getting back up to my bed on the second floor. I was so disheartened. All I could still seemingly do, was sleep and rest. Everything else taxed my body beyond its physical capabilities.

As time passed, my joy became walking Brodi, my cairn terrier, for 5 minutes a day. There were many days however, when the walk had to remain for another day, I was simply too exhausted and weak. On the days that I was able to go for a walk with her however, the walk proved to be quite a challenge as I struggled with muscle trembling and weakness, burning in my thighs, painful spasms in my back, heart palpitations, uncertainty in the placement of my feet and labored breathing. I frequently had to stop and sit along the way to catch my breath, regain my strength and footing, and encourage myself – I could do this! Getting back home was a difficult pursuit but my bed awaited me, and it would magically alleviate many of my symptoms. Over time, my incessant need for sleep was replaced by my incessant need for total, bed rest. Thankfully, I was experiencing some improvement and as time progressed, I moved from being mostly bedridden, to mostly housebound.

The numerous, varied, relentless and debilitating physical challenges of my disease experiences were very, concerning for me when it came to my little Brodi. Brodi, in many respects, is my little girl and she brings so much joy to my life. At the time of my diagnosis, she was only two years old and was brimming with energy, curiosity and adventure. Sadly, at such a young age, she had learned what "time to go to sleep" meant and would dutifully lie down by my side and sleep for hours on end with me. I am so thankful that Brodi is independent, intelligent and learned how to make her own fun. She would frequently jump up on the bed, flip her ball into the air and gleefully, jump off and make a mad dash to retrieve it. Many times, over the years, I envisioned Brodi putting a small packsack on her back, filled with her favorite treats and toys, and heading off down the road in search of a more physically active and interactive parent. I certainly did not have much to offer her and it hurt me deeply. To this day, I have no idea how parents with a more moderate to severe ME/CFS diagnosis do it. There were so many days when just the thought of feeding and putting Brodi out in the backyard were exhausting for me. I cannot fathom being responsible for a child's physical, cognitive and spiritual well-being, when one is struggling deeply with this disease. It must be very, heart wrenching for a parent!

Similarly, I have no doubt that ME/CFS can challenge the life that two people once lovingly shared together. I watched myself go from a physically and socially active individual to one who could barely meet the simplest of her life's demands. I was certainly, not the person who I once was – I required so much sleep, rest and solitude, and simple acts such as engaging in a short conversation could induce many symptoms including migraines, anxiety, frustration and irritability. I was so physically challenged by ME/CFS that I quite simply had no energy left for anyone or anything else including a smile, understanding and compassion. Being an active, loving and thoughtful partner was now, totally beyond my capabilities.

From my perspective, ME/CFS can be life changing for both partners and can impact even the most caring of relationships. My heart goes out to all those individuals who have or who are currently experiencing a chronic, invisible and debilitating disease in their life together.

In summation, my journey with ME/CFS involved an array of physical challenges, the most challenging of which was fatigue. The level of fatigue in my body was so profound that just the thought of movement or activity exhausted me even further. Any level of physical exertion, no matter how inconsequential, exacerbated my fatigue levels and intensified my numerous other symptoms. The fatigue and overall physical malaise made my life one, huge struggle and my inability to undertake even the simplest of things, was so soul diminishing. I felt like my entire life was on hold and that there was seemingly, nothing that I could do about it.

The frustration, sadness, disillusionment and disbelief that accompanied my physical debilitation were all too often, all too overpowering for me. I did not know where to turn, what to do or how to address my many, physical challenges. I felt lost, alone and broken, and unlike any previous life experience, I could not get back up and get back to my life. My usual modus operandi of sheer will power, determination and positive thinking seemed to be no match for ME/CFS. I was adrift and longed for home.

The physical challenges of ME/CFS have erased much of the life that I once lived and loved. My ability to play sports, to be socially active and to pursue my career, have all but disappeared. This disease has left me too exhausted and malaised to even think about pursuing the things that once filled my life with joy including, dreaming new dreams. My life is truly, a small semblance of what it once was and I am frequently, tormented by the loss of the person who I once saw myself as, the person who I believed I was – physically healthy, competent, vibrant and adventurous. Admittedly, there are times when I feel like I might be making a bit of progress, only to find myself back in bed, unable to do things for days at a time. Even after all these years, ME/CFS continues to drastically limit my life! I often question if my body is simply not ready to be "pushed" to do things or if this is the "new" extent of my physical capabilities – the new extent of my life's physical pursuits.

My cognitive challenges

ME/CFS posed numerous, varied, relentless and debilitating cognitive challenges for me as well. Among these challenges were a severely compromised ability to think, sustain attention, recall information, follow discussions and express my ideas. This made socializing with family and close friends, my only real social activity, very, difficult for me. I was so cognitively exhausted that I felt like my brain was operating in slow motion – I lived in a perpetual state of mental fog. I also had great difficulty focusing on the task at hand, processing simple information and reading, a passion of mine, had become a frustrating and demeaning experience. I had such difficulty concentrating on the text, following the ideas and remembering what I had just read. It was all so disheartening!

I was uncharacteristically, very forgetful and constantly misplacing things. I would for example, go to do something and within seconds, I forgot what I was intending to do or, I would have something in my hand one moment and the next, I could not find it. It was as though the object, like my thoughts, had evaporated into thin air. I was also no longer able to multi-task, something that I was previously adept at. Attempting to multi-task only left me confused, disoriented, anxious and frustrated. Furthermore, I was always making mistakes. Wrapping Christmas gifts for example, which was typically a very happy occasion for me, was wrought with mistakes, impatience and utter frustration. First, I lacked the physical energy to round up the paper and bows from the basement and secondly, I lacked the cognitive energy and acuity necessary to make the correct paper measurements. For some reason, I kept making mistakes with the wrapping paper's size requirements, over-and-over-and-over again. My problem-solving skills were clearly, sorely lacking as well! Moreover, my psychomotor skills were severely compromised. My fingers for example, seemed to no longer do what I needed them to do. Something as simple as using scissors or trying to screw a nut on a bolt were really challenging for me. It was as though the messaging between my fingers and brain was lacking, as though my fingers and brain were now two totally, separate operating systems, choosing to disregard any messaging from the other while, I sat in the middle wondering what was happening. There was such a paucity in my thoughts and movements, a huge open space where nothing was seemingly happening. It was surreal! Once again, I had to push myself hard, constantly tell myself that I could do this and often, I had to walk away – frustrated, exhausted and needing hours of sleep. What were once easy and joyful experiences, were now almost impossible undertakings – they were so beyond my cognitive capabilities.

In addition, I struggled to think, my thoughts were always, muddled and the processing of information was no longer done with ease. In fact, my thinking, information processing and decision-making abilities were severely compromised. I found myself struggling for example, to make sense of new information, identify a logical path forward and make a sound decision. I increasingly, found myself having to rely on family and close friends for their feedback and advice – I was so cognitively inept and incapable of making a good decision. I am very grateful that they were there for me, patiently listening and letting me pass my ideas by them. Their advice and counsel gave me comfort, allayed my fears and anxiety, and provided me with the confidence to move forward with my decisions. This once confident, independent and fairly, successful woman was now struggling with and second guessing everything about her thinking and decision-making processes. I felt inadequate and lost in so many aspects of my life and my self-esteem, self-confidence and self-identity really started to take a beating.

Living in a perpetual state of mental fog and cognitive ineptness made simple things, like leaving the house to go and pick up a few groceries, a real struggle for me. As I drove down the road and approached the store, I could feel my self-doubt and anxiety mounting over my "new" cognitive reality. Once at the store, to conserve my physical energy, I would often ask an employee where I might find the product that I was looking for. So often, I could not think of the product's name, nor describe its use. My words and mental images, no matter how desperately I tried, eluded me. Paying for the grocery items was no small feat either. Focusing on the amount of money that I owed, taking out the right number of bills, trying to remember how much I had given the cashier, and trying to calculate what change I might expect back were impossible undertakings. My brain was no longer able to perform these functions. Trying to recall my credit card PIN number was a whole other matter (and no, there was no tap function at the time). Everything in my life was arduous and I increasingly, felt physically and cognitively inept. As I previously noted, I had to adapt to my "new" life circumstances so, I started to shop on the internet and in small, convenience stores. The internet and convenience stores became my go to places as they required far less of my depleted cognitive and physical energy levels, reduced my high levels of self-doubt and anxiety, and were much less, demeaning experiences for me.

Socializing with family and close friends was extremely, cognitively challenging for me as well. Our time together demanded a cognitive energy and adeptness that I no longer had. My mental acuity was so sorely lacking that even with the greatest of intent, I struggled to sustain my attention, follow the conversation, process what they were saying and find the words to express my ideas. Often, in the middle of a sentence, I would also forget what I was talking about. The simple acts of attentively listening, processing and recalling information and participating in a conversation, were now extremely challenging, totally exhausting and very humiliating for me. By the end of our visits, I was filled with high levels of anxiety, frustration, discouragement and embarrassment over my cognitive inadequacies, and required endless hours of sleep for days after. I recall thinking, I once had the cognitive capacity to complete a Ph.D. but now, I cannot actively participate in a conversation with family and close friends. My life felt so shattered! On many occasions, I wondered if I would ever recover and be the person who I once enjoyed being, the person who loved to engage in conversations, share new ideas and spend time with family and friends. I was extremely, disheartened by my "new" cognitive reality.

Visits with close friends could be disheartening from another perspective. Our time together often left me with a more heightened awareness of my physical and cognitive shortcomings and shone a bright light on how ME/CFS had debilitated and drastically changed my life. While I love to share time with my friends and hear about their successes, adventures and the new people in their life, our conversations could be painful for me. While they continued to embrace and be full participants in their lives, I could not and as hard as I tried, I could not get back to the life that I once loved and actively shared with them. I felt so beaten by my "new" life. The frustration and deep sorrow over my severely compromised physical and cognitive abilities could be overwhelming, and added even more, to the burden of living with ME/CFS.

Receiving telephone calls from former colleagues and managers were also difficult for me. As much as I loved to hear from them, I was riddled with anxiety over my cognitive inadequacies. I once again, had to struggle to sustain my attention, recall information and find the words to express my ideas. Moreover, I did not want them to know what had become of me, how shattered my life was. At that point in time, I was reluctant to share my diagnosis, as ME/CFS sounded like a rather benign disorder and in no way, conveyed the devastating effects that this disease was having on my life. Furthermore, I could not adequately explain what ME/CFS was nor what might have caused it. Following our conversations, I would also find myself second guessing everything that had transpired. I questioned whether I had conveyed the necessary information coherently and accurately, whether they sensed my anxiety, frustration and brokenness, and whether they might judge me for any mistakes that I might have made. What was once a pleasant and confident exchange with people I cared about was now extremely taxing, riddled with uncertainty and anxiety, and so soul diminishing for me. These calls took so much from me, on so many levels!

Any cognitive requirement would further intensify my cognitive fatigue and precipitate other symptoms such as dizziness, nausea, weakness, disorientation and migraines. I was so cognitively challenged by ME/CFS that, after a while, I opted to run on auto pilot. Thinking took energy, energy that I no longer had. This led to some now, quite laughable situations. At the time however, I did not find these events to be so funny. I recall for example, arriving at my sister's place in my very comfortable but tattered slippers. It was only when I stepped into her house and went to take off my shoes that I realized I was out and about town, in my slippers. My sister and brother-in-law greeted me with a surprised look on their faces and my sister asked me if I was ok. It was so uncharacteristic of me – never, before had this happened. I was just not thinking! Not long thereafter, I found myself in the middle of a convenience store once again, with my old, unappealing slippers on. Clearly, this whole auto pilot stuff was not working either!

In summation, my journey with ME/CFS has been plagued by numerous and relentless cognitive challenges. The most challenging of which, was living in a perpetual state of cognitive exhaustion and mental fog. I had to slowly pick my way through my mental world. I was uncharacteristically, forgetful, constantly making mistakes and misplacing things, and had great difficulty problem-solving and making sound decisions. Socializing with family and close friends, something that was previously done with great ease and much joy, was now done under much duress and frustration. In many respects, my cognitive life was reduced to struggling with the simple acts of thinking, talking and performing the most modest of motor skills. It was so demeaning and all too often, much too overwhelming for me. Moreover, any amount of cognitive activity intensified my physical and cognitive fatigue levels further and triggered so many, other symptoms. There was absolutely, no escaping the relentless cognitive challenges nor their debilitating effects on my life.

The cognitive exhaustion and ineptness dogged everything that I did and filled my life with high levels of frustration, anxiety, irritability and despair. They also caused me to struggle with my self-confidence, self-esteem and self-identity. I was deeply discouraged and distraught and frequently, sat in a state of disbelief. I just wanted to cry, my life felt so shattered and I, once again, did not know where to turn nor how to pull my life together. The fairly, intelligent and competent individual who I once believed l was, was no longer apparent to me – the person who stood before me in the mirror was unrecognizable! My cognitive challenges tormented me on many levels and I frequently found myself wondering if this was the "new" extent of my cognitive capabilities. This was such an inconceivable notion and yet increasingly, appeared to be my "new" cognitive reality, my "new" norm.

My spiritual challenges

According to the World Health Organization (WHO) "spiritual health refers to that part of the individual which reaches out and strives for meaning and purpose in life. It is the intangible "something" that transcends physiology and psychology" [5]. Indicators of spiritual health include a connection with others, oneself, nature and God [6]. Spiritual health relates to an individual's values, beliefs and faith, and contributes to one's overall physical, mental and social well-being [5].

I am typically, a person who tries to rise to a challenge and face life head on. ME/CFS however, on many occasions, has left me wanting to pull the blankets over my head and let the world go by. Not because I did not want to deal with my life but rather, I was too physically, cognitively and spiritually exhausted to do so. I felt like I had nothing left in me to get up with and nothing left in me to offer others. My usual strong resolve was gone, my mind over matter belief was adrift and my belief in the God who I had come to believe in was waning. In many respects, I felt like core aspects of my "way of being" in the world, my spiritual well-being, was slowly being stripped away. Of all my ME/CFS experiences, my spiritual challenges were the ones that most "rocked my world". They blew open my life in terms of how I saw myself in relation to others, to myself and to my God. My spiritual challenges also caused me to struggle deeply with some of my long-held values, beliefs and religious principles.

Before my journey with ME/CFS, I would never have thought that a chronic and invisible disease could have such an impact on an individual's spiritual well-being, on an individual's "way of being" in the world. I firmly, believed that my "way of being" would withstand the tests of time but ME/CFS proved me wrong. An incident at a grocery store that really left me reeling, aghast and ashamed of myself illustrates this impact. I was in the check-out line and was physically struggling – I was dizzy, tired, in pain and needed to get home to bed. I was also anxious about my impaired cognitive abilities and frustrated by my life in general. The woman in front of me was simply counting her pennies and recounting her pennies. Yes, we still had pennies in Canada then! I remember thinking very unkind thoughts like "what the !!! is wrong with you, give the cashier the $20. bill that you have in your hand, put your pennies back in your purse and get the !!! out of here". I could not believe that these thoughts were mine and was very taken aback! It was not like me to be that irritable, judgmental and unkind in my thoughts towards others. I believe in the importance of kindness in my interactions

23

and of putting positive energy into the universe but now, I found myself struggling to just be civil. There were other, similar situations that left me questioning, at a very fundamental level, what was happening to me and who was I becoming? In addition to my many physical and cognitive struggles, my "way of being" in the world was now under siege!!

I also started to notice changes in my interactions with family and friends, people who I love very, deeply. I have always tried to be there for my family and friends and to help them in any way that I could. I now however, found myself impatient and irritable when I heard of their circumstances. I just wanted to shout "leave me alone, I don't care anymore! I have nothing left to give you! You made your choices." I was clearly, no longer able to weather the ups or downs of their life and was increasingly, becoming less empathetic and more judgmental towards their circumstances. This too, was uncharacteristic of me. In fact, I would never have believed that such thoughts towards my loved ones were even remotely, possible. But my help and support for them came at great cost to me. Hearing of their circumstances extracted so much from me, plummeting me further into physical, cognitive and spiritual exhaustion and malaise, leaving me feeling even more defeated and unable to cope with my own daily life.

I was increasingly, becoming a person whom I did not recognize nor want to be. I was uncharacteristically, living with anger, frustration, impatience, irritability, anxiety, despair, depression and disillusionment. I hated always being short-fused and on edge. I hated feeling like a wounded animal always ready to snarl and growl at the people and situations in my life. I hated that it was becoming ever harder for me to gain control over my emotions and regain some sense of spiritual well-being and connectedness. I was experiencing an irritability and impatience that made me want to run away from myself! It was as though a dragon lady had taken control of my way of being in the world. I once saw myself as a fairly, decent person who tried to extend kindness, compassion and understanding to others but now, I was struggling deeply to just be civil with them. This "new" disposition, this new "way of being" in the world, hurt me deeply – it was like a deep cut to my soul. I was increasingly, losing touch with my spiritual connectedness with others and with life itself. This saddened and concerned me deeply.

So many questions regarding this "new" disposition swirled around in my head. I wondered for example, why I could not regain my usual "way of being" in the world, my sense of connectedness and my sense of centeredness. I also wondered whether the unrelenting physical and cognitive challenges were so overwhelming that my body was taxed beyond its capabilities, wearing me down to the point of such rawness and finally, I questioned if this disease might take me to the point where I could not withstand anymore. Looking back, I suppose that I was struggling so deeply to just get through my days and coping so hard with my own life, that I really did not have anything left in me to offer others. In many respects, I felt like I had lost my true north – I was in such an unfamiliar place and my soul ached. I could not do, I could not think and now, I could not even be kind or be the person who I most wanted to be in this world. I was tormented on so many levels of my spiritual health. ME/CFS tested me to the core of my being and caused much spiritual distress.

I was also growing tired of having to constantly address "others'" misconceptions and judgements about me and this disease. Moreover, "others'" views were often difficult for me to come to terms with and caused me to struggle even further. I, consequently, began to distance myself. I understand, very well, that ME/CFS is not an easy disease to comprehend. I also understand that people generally, mean well. Their well-intentioned pep talks, comments on the improbability of me being so exhausted, suggestions on what I needed to do to heal myself and statements on how I should just push through things nonetheless, left me feeling alone, downtrodden and floundering. I often felt like I was not measuring up, like I was being judged and like I needed to constantly explain myself and this disease. I typically, do not just walk away from things and generally, have no problem sharing my experiences and points of view. In fact, I quite enjoy those exchanges. However, in this case, it was easier to distance myself because to do otherwise drained me physically, cognitively and spiritually, leaving me struggling all the more with my daily life. Moreover, I did not have the cognitive energy nor the mental acuity to discuss this complex, multisystem disease nor justify its devastating effects on my life.

Through time, when asked how I was doing, I simply responded "great". What was the point of talking about it? Saying everything was great was far less exhausting and in many respects, less demeaning than engaging in a conversation about my health status and what I should be doing about it. I sometimes thought, if a change of mind, pushing through it and healthy eating habits were all that were needed, I would have recovered already. Thankfully, my GP and psychologist understood how life changing this disease can be. They were a welcome refuge, a go to place of understanding, compassion, validation and sound counsel – something that my soul yearned for, so badly. In many regards, they watered my parched soul.

Unlike any previous illness experience, ME/CFS invited me perhaps, even forced me, to look deeply within and to travel to places that I may not have otherwise. ME/CFS asked me for example, to really look at myself and to consider my culpability in this disease – whether I might have brought it on by not sufficiently taking care of my health and whether I may have put other people's needs before my own health. ME/CFS also asked me to examine some of my religious beliefs – whether ME/CFS might have been karmic, whether it was life "haphazardly" happening or, if it was all a part of God's plan for me. Many of these questions initially, brought me back to my workplace. As noted earlier, prior to leaving my workplace and career because of ME/CFS, I had been working on a number of reorganizations over a 14-month period. After the third reorganization, deep down I knew that I could not sustain another one, not knowing that the 4th was imminent. I was extremely tired, had just had shoulder surgery and was in a fair amount of pain. I decided however, when hearing of the 4th reorganization, that I would push forward and give it my personal best.

As I reflected upon that timeframe, I found myself questioning if the emotional toll of caring deeply about the employees and managers, and having to constantly push myself through my tiredness and pain, might have contributed to the onset of this disease. I also pondered why I did not listen to my body and ask to be removed from the 4th reorganization – why did I choose to put other people's needs first particularly, in view of the exhaustion and physical pain that I was in? I further questioned if this illness might have been karmic. At point in time, I was open to any possible factor that might have contributed to my disease state. While my intentions were to help managers and employees through the reorganizations maybe, just maybe, being associated with the reorganizations created a negative, karmic energy, an energy that found its way back to my health. Finally, I wondered where my God was. The God that I believed in promises an abundant life – a life that includes good health. How then, could this have happened?

I struggled with many other questions as well such as, did this disease happen haphazardly and if so, what did that say about my faith? Is there a life lesson that I need to learn from this experience? If my health does not improve, what might my life be about moving forward, and can I find meaning in that life? I desperately searched for answers to these questions. In many respects, I felt like my life was falling apart, like the ground was constantly shifting under my feet, and like my life was crashing in on me. So many of my long-held values and beliefs were being brought into question. These questions tormented me and turned my life upside down and inside out. The "centeredness" that I once felt in my life was gone. I was struggling so deeply at the spiritual level that oft times, I felt like I was in the winter of my life – there was uncharacteristically such a darkness and malcontent. At times, all I could see was the desolation – my life and my "way of being" in the world had been so scorched by this disease. I experienced many dark days and nights of the soul with ME/CFS.

Many of the pillars that once sustained my life were also crumbling around me. The loss of my physical and cognitive abilities, my high energy levels, my stamina and athleticism, my determination, independence and will power, my optimism and self-confidence, my inner strength, my career, my ability to socialize and travel, my sense of adventure, my ability to read and write for hours, my ability to dream and look forward to better days, my spiritual well-being, my sense of joy and happiness in life, my gratitude for being alive and sadly, some friends. Things that once brought me great joy like children, animals, gardening and natural beauty were now being met with little emotion as well. Even spending time with my great nephews and nieces, whom I adore, left me saddened. I simply did not have the energy to actively participate in their lives through play and sports and some days, not even to sit and chat with them. The fire in my soul was so badly diminished.

I once took such joy in physical movement, in intellectual and spiritual pursuits, in feeling connected to life and in embracing my esprit de corps. I once ran to life with open arms and much vigor but with ME/CFS, I no longer had the energy to do, think, feel or run to anyone or anything. My essence appeared to have been extinguished. ME/CFS stripped away so much that I felt like a bystander in my own life! For such a previously active person, who once lovingly and joyfully embraced her life, these losses were difficult to come to terms with. A very, deep sense of loss hounded me. Things that I never thought I could lose, were no longer a part of my life. I often felt like all the goodness and joy had been sucked from my life.

At times, the sadness and despair over what my life had become, the many losses that I faced and the person who I was becoming, were all too much to deal with. I was also increasingly, becoming tired of having to constantly cope and remain positive – trying to spin all of this in a more positive light. In those moments, I wondered if ME/CFS might break my spirit – if this disease might take me to the point where I no longer had any fight left in me and where I no longer cared about anyone or anything. Sitting with these emotions and thoughts scared me. While I knew that I had to acknowledge and address them, I was also cognizant of not allowing myself to go too deeply into them. I frequently, felt like there was a "big, black hole" beckoning me and that should I enter it, I might not be able to come back out. I would be totally, consumed by it! There were other times, when I would hear my inner voice say "I don't want to live like this anymore, I just want to die". At those moments, I questioned if my spirit was approaching the breaking point. At a deeper level however, I knew that no matter how bad things got, no matter how much despair I might be in, I needed to choose life. Even when I felt like I could no longer tread water, I knew that I needed to get to the shoreline. I needed to get to that place inside of me that would always choose to move forward, even if it was a matter of simply and slowly, putting one foot before the other. My spirit though downtrodden, was thankfully still alive. In the depths of this despair, I could certainly relate to why ME/CFS patients experience higher rates of depression and suicide, as will be discussed in Chapter 5. ME/CFS required me to dig deep and to cling to the hope of better days to come.

In summation, as with my physical and cognitive challenges, my spiritual challenges were equally numerous, unrelenting and devastating. In many respects, my spiritual challenges rocked my world and turned my life upside down and inside out. So much so, that I felt I no longer knew who I was nor what I believed in. ME/CFS caused me to struggle deeply with many of my long-held values and beliefs including, how I saw myself in the world, who I was in relation to others and who my God was. My "way of being" in the world, my spiritual well-being, was being stripped away by ME/CFS. I frequently prayed that there would be some resolve to my spiritual challenges and that I would, once again, joyfully experience spiritual health and well-being.

Figure 1: Maslow's Hierarchy of Needs

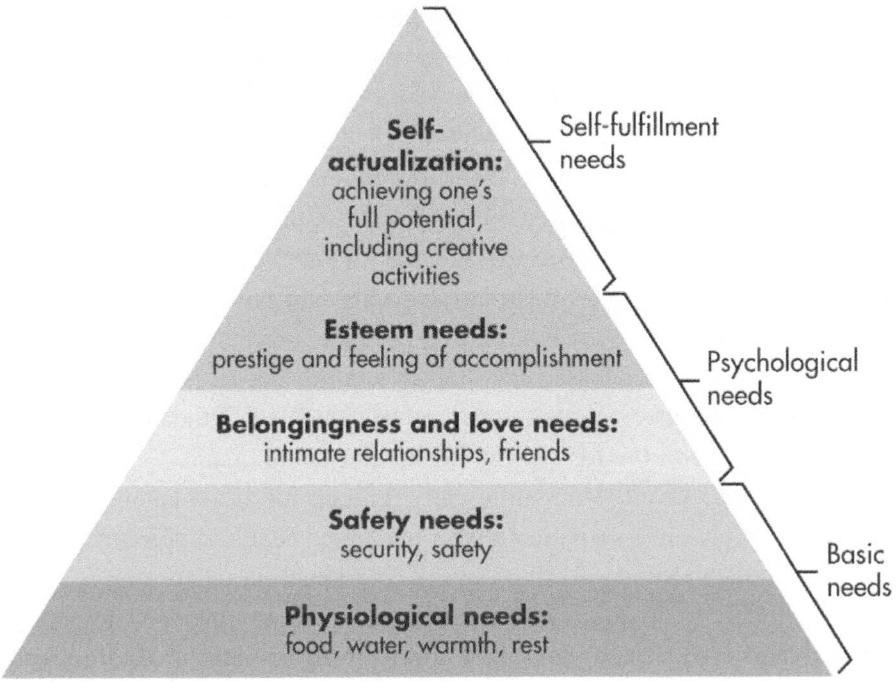

Sources: https://en.wikipedia.org/wiki/Maslow'shierarchyofneeds and www.simplypsychology.org/maslow

Before concluding this chapter, I would like to add that on many occasions throughout my journey with ME/CFS, I found myself thinking about Maslow's hierarchy of needs. I suppose I was trying to put some context around my physical, cognitive and spiritual experiences. As you may recall, Maslow identified 5 levels of human need (Figure 1). The most basic of these levels are the physiological level or, the human need for food, water, warmth and rest and the safety level or, the need for physical safety and security. The third and fourth levels, the psychological needs levels, speak to the human needs of belongingness, love and a sense of accomplishment. The fifth and final level, self-actualization, is the individuals' need to achieve their full potential. ME/CFS had clearly, left me struggling at the most basic of all human needs, that of the physiological and safety needs levels. Quite simply, I had no energy to pursue any of the other needs' levels. As noted earlier, attempting to socialize with family and close friends or level 3 belongingness needs, extracted a heavy toll on my already, depleted energy levels. In many respects, I was too tired to belong! And, forget about fulfilling my sense of accomplishment or achieving my full potential (levels 4 and 5) – I was so exhausted and malaised that these needs were sadly, non-existent. I was too tired to even dream a dream!

In terms of meeting my levels one and two needs, I discovered that I was very, fortunate. Given the severity of my ME/CFS disease state, I was no longer able to work in any capacity and will be forever thankful that I had an employee benefit plan. Unlike so many other ME/CFS patients, as will be discussed in Chapter 5, I did not have to struggle to maintain a steady income, a roof over my head or food on the table. Facing and struggling with the loss of my health and being unable to return to a workplace that I loved, were sufficiently difficult for me. I cannot fathom the illness experience of patients who lose their health, employment and financial independence. To find oneself in a situation where one is so ill and yet, unable to do anything but sleep and rest, and quietly watch one's finances and hard-earned gains go to ruins, must be very devastating and demoralizing. I have no hesitation in saying that my physical, cognitive and spiritual health would have been even more negatively impacted, had I struggled with the loss of my income, home and financial independence.

My heart goes out to all of those individuals who suffer from ME/CFS or other chronic illnesses and who, as a result of their disease experience, face a reduced or total loss of income and have no other financial means of supporting themselves. This must make an already difficult situation, all the more intolerable.

In summation, the physical, cognitive and spiritual challenges that I experienced on my ME/CFS journey, as depicted in Table 1, were numerous, varied, relentless, debilitating and life changing. Each of these three "challenge areas" have made my ME/CFS journey a difficult one. The accumulation of the numerous and debilitating symptoms from all three of these "challenge areas", acting in tandem, however, have made my daily life even more challenging, complex and burdensome. Simple activities, like working in my garden for example, were met with extreme physical and cognitive fatigue, excruciating body pain, nose bleeds, trembling in my hands, muscle spasms, heat intolerance, labored breathing, heart palpitations, pain in my left chest, nausea, dizziness, compromised psychomotor skills, cognitive ineptness, and anguish, frustration, irritability and despair. The disease state, as a result of the accumulation of the varied and debilitating symptoms from the three "challenge areas", acting in tandem, almost defies description it was so overwhelming and life limiting.

Table 1: A summary of my physical, cognitive and spiritual challenges

Physical Challenges	Cognitive Challenges	Spiritual Challenges
• debilitating fatigue/ extreme exhaustion • worsening of symptoms following physical, cognitive or spiritual exertion • hip, jaw, muscle, joint and abdominal pain, feet and hand stiffness, morning stiffness, migraines	• extreme cognitive exhaustion, lived in a perpetual state of mental fog • severely compromised ability to think, recall information, process information, express ideas and make decisions • slower cognitive processes, problem	• overwhelmed by life's simplest of demands and difficulty coping with daily life • mood disorders – anxiety, irritability, impatience, despair, depression, disillusionment, sadness, frustration, anger • reduced ability to dream and be optimistic about the future

Physical Challenges	Cognitive Challenges	Spiritual Challenges
• severe muscle spasms in back, neck and legs • trembling in hands, arms and legs • pressure in the head, nose bleeds, nausea, dizziness, light headedness, overall weakness • difficulty falling and staying asleep • dry eyes, blurred vision, earaches, sore lymph nodes • irritable bowel, urinary frequency • heart palpitations, numbness in the face, legs and arms, chest pain, panic attacks • sensitivities to light, noise, smell, food and medications • intolerances to heat and cold • night chills and sweats • more severe flues and increased sensitivities to vaccines • hair loss and changes in skin pigmentation • no physical stamina	solving difficulties and short-term memory loss • attention deficits and concentration difficulties • uncharacteristically forgetful and constantly making mistakes/ misplacing things • impaired coordination/ psychomotor skills • slowed reaction times and balance problems • disoriented when standing, walking and when confronted with loud noises and bright lights • inability to multi-task • difficulty engaging in conversations and socializing	• deep sense of loss and brokenness • changes in my "ways of being" (e.g., nothing left to offer others, unkind in my thoughts towards others, withdrew from others) • mental anguish and social isolation • felt alone and misunderstood • loss of self-confidence, self-esteem and self-identity • questioned and reassessed personal beliefs, values and religious principles • reduced sense of spiritual well-being and connectedness

In concluding this chapter, ME/CFS brought my life to an abrupt halt. For the first 12 months or so, for all intents and purposes, I was bedridden. This disease left me barely able to move, think or be the person who I most wanted to be. For the longest time, my life was totally consumed by the simplest of my life's demands. It took everything that I had to feed myself, to stand and walk, to talk with others and to care for Brodi. ME/CFS stripped away so much from my life! A life that I once passionately embraced and joyfully lived, began to feel so foreign to me. ME/CFS scorched my previous life beyond recognition and as hard as I tried, I did not seem to have any influence over this disease nor its devastating effects on my life.

ME/CFS tormented me on the physical, cognitive and spiritual levels of my being and has challenged me to my core. So many times, over the years, I have sat in disbelief at the state of my life. Everything that I attempted to do, no matter how nominal, was like a mirror reflecting my physical, cognitive and spiritual ineptness and brokenness. There has been no escaping the very, heavy burden of this disease. I have frequently found myself wondering if I would ever regain some semblance of the life that I once passionately lived and loved. If I would ever again, be an active and happy participant in my life. My world, once vibrant and rich with color sadly, had become dull and opaque. To move forward, ME/CFS asked me to dig deep and find the strength within.

In my quest to understand my varied physical, cognitive and spiritual challenges and their devastating and life changing effects on my life, I turned to the research literature and thankfully, found answers therein. Chapter 3 will explore some of the research findings that have helped me to understand this complex disease and my many experiences with it.

Chapter 3

SO, WHAT IS ME/CFS AND HOW DOES IT MANIFEST ITSELF?

Find a place inside where there's joy, and the joy will burn out the pain
~ Joseph Campbell

Life is full of happiness and tears; be strong and have faith
~ Kareena Kapoor Khan

When I received my ME/CFS diagnosis, I had little understanding of this disease, its range of symptoms, causes, severity, risk factors and treatments. Quite simply, I had no goal posts by which to understand, assess or address my relentless and devastating physical, cognitive and spiritual challenges with this disease.

It was only deep within the research literature that I began to understand that I was living with a complex disease of no known cause. Moreover, ME/CFS consists of a fairly, broad spectrum of disease severity, numerous, varied and debilitating symptoms, and overlapping medical conditions that can complicate the patients' disease state. This chapter will seek to shed some light on this chronic, invisible and devastating disease by providing an overview and definition of ME/CFS. It will also discuss the risk factors, possible causes, how a diagnosis is rendered, and the various case definitions/criteria. Finally, it will discuss the overlapping medical conditions and how the severity of the disease is graded. All of these, more "general" topics, helped me to cobble together a more fulsome understanding of ME/CFS and my experiences with it.

The origins of the term ME/CFS

ME/CFS is not a new phenomenon and has been causing suffering since the 1850s. At that point in time, the disorder was referred to as neurasthenia or nervous exhaustion, a psychological disorder. The major symptom of this disorder was a long-lasting fatigue. In the 1930s, 1950s and 1980's, outbreaks of a similar, long-lasting and disabling fatigue were again reported [1, 2, 3].

The term myalgic encephalomyelitis (ME) is used to identify this disease in many countries throughout the world most particularly, in Europe. This term refers to *my* – muscle, *algic* – pain, *encephalo* – brain, *myel* – spinal cord and *itis* – inflammation. In 1969, the term benign myalgic encephalomyelitis was classified into the International Classification of Diseases under a disease of the nervous system [2, 3, 4]. Over time, ME has become associated more with muscle pain, muscle fatigability, overall fatigue and extraordinary symptom fluctuation rather than, a psychological disorder [4].

Chronic fatigue syndrome (CFS), on the other hand, is commonly used to identify this disease in North America. CFS was first characterized by extreme fatigue and was associated with symptoms such as, headaches, sore throat, lymph node pain and myalgia [4]. In 1987, this disease, described as a condition resembling the Epstein Barr Virus (EBV), more commonly known as mononucleosis, was presented in the medical literature [4]. In 1988, the term CFS replaced EBV [5]. As fatigue is but one of the symptoms of this disorder, the term ME/CFS is used as it "more accurately reflect(s) the complex nature of the condition" [6].

Over the years, ME/CFS has been referred to in a variety of ways including, chronic fatigue immune dysfunction syndrome (CFIDS), chronic epstein barr virus (EBV), post viral fatigue syndrome (PVFS), Akureyri disease, chronic infectious mononucleosis, epidemic neuromyasthenia, Iceland disease, myalgic encephalitis and most recently, as systemic exertion intolerance disease (SEID) [4, 7].

Some researchers have posited that the way in which an illness is labelled affects the patients' illness experience. They argue that labels convey meaning to both the patients and "others" in their world (e.g., family members, employers and medical personnel) [8]. This meaning can affect the patients' perceptions of the illness and so too, the perceptions and reactions of "others" to the patients' condition [9]. In 2015, the Committee on the Diagnostic Criteria for Myalgic Encephalomyelitis/Chronic Fatigue Syndrome, believing that the term ME/CFS might stigmatize patients and trivialize their medical disorder, recommended that the term systemic exertion intolerance disease (SEID) be used. The committee members suggested that SEID "captures the fact that exertion of any sort – physical, cognitive, emotional – can adversely affect these patients in many of their organ systems and in many aspects of their lives" [10]. The term systemic is intended to imply that the condition affects many body systems while exertion intolerance implies the central feature of the disease. The term disease, on the other hand, is intended to imply that there is a pathological mechanism underlying the condition, even though the cause of the disease and disease process remain unknown [11]. As noted in the Preface, while this disease has been referred to in a variety of ways over the years, the term ME/CFS has been used most consistently in North America and is increasingly, being used worldwide [11, 12]. In light of this, the term ME/CFS is being used throughout this book.

Definitions of ME/CFS

Over the years, ME/CFS has been defined in a variety of ways including "a serious, chronic, complex, multisystem disease … (that) dramatically limits the activities of affected patients. In its most severe form, this disease can consume the lives of those whom it afflicts" [13]. It has further been defined as a "pathophysiological, multi-system illness that occurs in both sporadic and epidemic forms" [14] and as "a syndrome of persistent incapacitating weakness or fatigue, accompanied by nonspecific somatic symptoms, lasting at least 6 months and not attributed to any known cause" [15]. Finally, it has been defined as "a complex, fluctuating condition characterized by emotional, mental and physical fatigue" [16] and as a "devastating, multi-system disease that causes dysfunction of the neurological, immune, endocrine and energy/metabolism systems" [17].

ME/CFS has further been described as an "enigmatic and poorly recognized clinical entity" [18], a complex syndrome of enigmatic origin [19] and a debilitating and complex disorder that is characterized by profound fatigue [20]. It has also been described as a "physiological and biological disorder that is associated with multiple pathophysiological changes, that effect multiple body systems" [21]. Finally, ME/CFS has been described as a profound, debilitating fatigue that is long lasting. This fatigue can result in a substantial reduction in the individuals' personal, occupational, social and educational status [22].

The risk factors for ME/CFS

ME/CFS is an indiscriminate disease. It afflicts males and females, and people of all age groups including children, all racial and ethnic groups, and all social strata [1, 5, 23, 24].

ME/CFS typically, occurs between the ages of 30 and 50. It thus, tends to afflict the more highly functioning and productive members of the population [22]. Women are 2 to 4 times more likely than men to develop this disease and an estimated 60-85% of all patients are women between the ages of 40-59 [5, 3]. Some researchers posit that the increased rates in women may be associated with early menopause and other gynecological conditions such as endometriosis [3, 5]. There is no direct evidence to suggest that ME/CFS is contagious. However, blood relatives of people with ME/CFS may be more predisposed to this disease [23]. In fact, one study found that 73% of all patients had first degree relatives (i.e., father, mother, siblings) diagnosed with ME/CFS and 35% had first degree relatives diagnosed with an auto immune disorder such as Crohn's [25].

In Canada, over half a million Canadians (Table 2), aged 12 and over, or 1.9% of the total Canadian population, have been diagnosed with ME/CFS [26]. By comparison, in 2014, approximately 408,000 Canadians or 1.4% of the Canadian population reported a diagnosis, 63% of whom were women. Over the 2012 and 2014 timeframe, the number of Canadians reporting a diagnosis remained fairly, stable. The substantial, 37% increase in the number of Canadians reporting a diagnosis over the 2014-2017 time period [26], may be due to an increase in the number of patients being diagnosed, patients being more comfortable reporting their diagnosis or possibly, reporting changes.

Table 2: Number of Canadians reporting a ME/CFS diagnosis, as a percentage of the total Canadian population aged 12 and older, 2012-2017

ME/CFS	2012	% of Popu.	2014	% of Popu.	2017 (**)	% of Popu. (**)
Total	411,562	1.4	407,789	1.4	560,000	1.9
Male	138,082 (33%)	1.0	149,013 (37%)	1.0		
Female	273,480 (67%)	1.9	258,776 (63%)	1.7		

Sources: Canadian Community Health Survey (2012 and 2014) https://www150.statca.gc.ca/n1/daily-quotidien/150617/t002b and https://www150.statcan.gc.ca/n1/daily-quotidien/150617/dq150617b.(**) Canadian Institute of Health Research (2018) [26].

In delving a little more deeply into the Canadian data for other possible risk factors (Table 3), one notes that approximately 390,000 Canadians, aged 25 and older, have been diagnosed with ME/CFS, 63% of whom were women. In terms of the age groups that are most afflicted by this disease, 54% were between the ages of 25 and 59, and 66% were between the ages of 45 and 74. In terms of educational level, individuals with post-secondary and more than post-secondary education were almost equally divided at 51% and 48%, respectively. In terms of household income, 61% were in the lowest two income quintiles perhaps, due to the loss of income that is typically, associated with this disease (as will be discussed in Chapter 5). Finally, 56% were married or living common law while, 77% reported white as their cultural identity. In short, Canadians who reported a ME/CFS diagnosis were women, between the ages of 45 and 74, had lower household incomes, were married or living common law, and were white.

Table 3: Prevalence of ME/CFS in Canada by selected characteristics, for the household population aged 25 and older, 2014

Selected Characteristics	Canadian Population with ME/CFS
Total population diagnosed	389,900
a) Sex:	
Men	145,800 (37%)
Women	244,200 (63%)
b) Age group	
25-44	86,900 (22%)
45-59	123,800 (32%)
60-74	131,700 (34%)
75+	47,700 (12%)
c) Highest level of education*	
Post-secondary	197,700 (51%)
More than post-secondary	184,900 (48%)
d) Household income	
1 – Lowest quintile	149,800 (38%)
2	91,100 (23%)
3	60,400 (16%)
4	50,000 (13%)
5 – Highest quintile	37,800 (10%)
e) Marital status*	
Married/common law	217,800 (56%)
Widowed/separated/divorced	93,000 (24%)
Never married	75,800 (20%)

Selected Characteristics	Canadian Population with ME/CFS
f) Cultural identity*	
White	297,700 (77%)
Non-white	70,100 (18%)

Source: 2014 Canadian Community Health Survey, https://www150.statcan.gc.ca/n1/daily-quotidien/150617/dq150617b. *does not total the Canadian population figure of 389,900

The possible causes of this disease

While a large body of research literature exists, there remains no known cause for this disease. Among the possible causes are viruses, infections, immune dysfunction, chemical toxins, environmental pollutants, neuroendocrine or hypothalamic-pituitary-adrenal axis (HPA) abnormalities, dysfunctions of the central nervous system, reduced cortisol levels, impaired exercise capacity, sleep disruptions, genetic constitution, stress, personality traits and psychological factors such as, emotional trauma and post-traumatic stress disorder (PTSD) [3, 7, 20]. Other possible causes include parasites, a previous illness such as mononucleosis, abnormal blood cell shape, abnormally low blood pressure, hypoglycemia, irritable bowel syndrome, allergies, surgery, anesthetics, immunizations and brain abnormalities [1, 3]. Interestingly, a recent study found that the top five causes of ME/CFS onset were infections (64%), stressful incidents at work or at home (39%), exposure to environmental toxins (20%), international travel (20%) and domestic travel (19%) [25].

It is further theorized however, that a combination of factors such as neurological, physiological, psychological and immunological may all be at play, to varying degrees, in the development of ME/CFS [27]. A variety of illnesses and conditions such as viruses, infections, stress, a genetic predisposition, age, prior illness and brain abnormalities may all act together, to varying degrees, in the development of this disease [3, 7]. Other research similarly suggests that ME/CFS may be caused by a convergence of physical, neurological, emotional and behavioral factors, all acting together. For example, a serious physical illness (e.g., a chronic viral infection) or an emotional event (e.g., a depression), may converge and interact with neurological issues (e.g., brain abnormalities) or genetic abnormalities (e.g., immune system dysfunction) and trigger the disease, in some patients [28].

One review of the research literature identified an astounding, 80 factors as possible causes of this disease. These factors were subsequently, categorized into five main groupings as follows: genetic defects, immune system abnormalities, infectious diseases and viruses, central nervous system and hormonal imbalances, and psychological factors and personality traits [3, 22]. In attempting to better understand how these possible causes might play a role in the development of ME/CFS, I delved a little more deeply into the research literature. In the following paragraphs, I would like to briefly discuss some of the findings, under these five main groupings, that were of interest to me.

Under the genetic defects grouping, I discovered that some individuals may actually, be born with a predisposition to ME/CFS. The genes associated with low blood pressure for example, may have something to do with the onset of ME/CFS in some patients [2]. Yet other genetic research suggests that the sympathetic nervous system, which controls the body's response to trauma, injury or other stressful events, may be at play in triggering the disease in individuals who have a predisposition to it [2, 3, 24]. Finally, abnormalities in patients' muscles and immunological responses to exercise may be other possible causes [29].

In terms of immune system abnormalities, the poor early control of infections or insults to the body caused by allergies to food, pollution or sensitivities to heavy metals for example, may predispose some patients to ME/CFS [3, 5, 23]. These abnormalities or auto-immune deficiencies may cause the immune system to either overreact or underreact to the infections or insults, leading to chronic inflammatory responses and eventually, to the disease state [3, 5, 23]. Events such as immunizations, anesthetics, and surgical and physical trauma may also be responsible for triggering the disease in some individuals [3]. In fact, 10% of all patients reported that their ME/CFS onset was associated with a medical injection and 8% with surgery [25]. Reduced cortisol levels, which relax constraints on the inflammatory and immune cell activation processes, may also trigger ME/

CFS [30]. It remains unclear however, if the immune system impairments are sufficient in themselves to trigger ME/CFS [31].

Under the grouping of infectious diseases and viruses, an estimated 80% of all ME/CFS cases start suddenly with an infection such as a cold, flu, upper respiratory issue, Q fever or lyme disease [3, 11]. Viruses such as the Epstein Barr (EBV), commonly known as mononucleosis, the human T cell lymphotropic virus (HTLV) and the Ross River Virus are also thought to be possible causes. In fact, the EBV is believed to lead to post infection conditions that cause 10-12% of all ME/CFS cases [3, 20]. Patients who experience a more severe case of EBV in their youth, may also be more likely to go on to develop ME/CFS later in their life [5]. The xenotropic murine leukemia related virus (XMRV), found in 67% of patients in one study, may be another possible cause [32] as is, the MLV-like virus which was found in 86.5% of patients in another study [33]. Finally, infections and viruses are believed to be responsible for both the invitation and persistence of ME/CFS [34]. While infections and viruses may be responsible for the disease activity in some patients, to date, no conclusive link has been found [3, 5].

In terms of the central nervous system and hormonal imbalances, many patients have been found to have abnormal levels of certain hormones in their body. Notably, abnormally high levels of serotonin, deficiencies of dopamine and insufficient levels of cortisol. These hormones, which are produced in the hypothalamus-pituitary-adrenal axis (HPA), control important body functions such as stress response, the sleep-wake cycle, motor control and depression [2, 6]. Increased levels of the neuropeptide Y, which are released following a stressful event, may also be linked to the dysfunction of the HPA axis. The increased levels of neuropeptide Y have in fact, been correlated with patients' ME/CFS symptom severity [12]. Again, it remains unclear if the central nervous system and hormonal imbalances are sufficient in themselves to trigger this disease [6].

Psychological factors such as the accumulation of exposure to life's stresses including, psychological distress [35], trauma during childhood [36] and post-traumatic stress disorder (PTSD) [35], may also be related to the disease onset in some patients. It is theorized that the accumulation of exposure to life's stresses may be factors in the pathology of ME/CFS, due to their effect on the immune, central nervous and neuroendocrine systems [35, 37]. Finally, in terms of personality traits, traits such as maladaptive perfectionism, defined as an excessive conscientiousness, may put some individuals at increased risk for developing ME/CFS. It is theorized that the increased levels of anxiety and tension that are typically, associated with excessive conscientiousness, in combination with the patients' own unique biological factors, may trigger ME/CFS in some individuals [38]. While personality traits may increase some individuals' susceptibility to the disease, they are believed to play only a minor role in the development of the disease [37, 39, 40]. Increasingly, ME/CFS is believed to be caused by metabolic, immunological and neurological abnormalities [41]. Figure 2 summarizes some of the possible causes of ME/CFS, by the five main groupings.

Figure 2: A visual summary of some of the possible causes of ME/CFS, by main grouping

Genetic defects	Immune system abnormalities	Infectious diseases and viruses
• Genetic constitution • Immune system dysfunction • Low blood pressure, hypoglycemia • Impaired exercise capacity, muscle abnormalities	• Autoimmune • Environmental pollutants, allergies • Surgical and physical trauma, anaesthetics, vaccinations	• Colds, flus, lyme disease, Q-fever • Epstein Barr Virus, xenotropic murine leukemia virus (XMRV), Ross River Virus

Central nervous system and hormonal imbalances	Psychological factors and personality traits
• Dysfunction of the hypothalamic-pituitary-adrenal axis (e.g., sleep dysfunction) • Hormone abnormalities (e.g., serotonin, dopamine, cortisol, neuropeptide Y)	• Accumulation of exposure to life's stresses • Emotional trauma, post traumatic stress disorder • Maladaptive perfectionism

Source: IACFS/ME (2012) [12] and research cited in this chapter.

Diagnosing ME/CFS

Diagnosing ME/CFS is not always an easy task for medical practitioners as there is no generally accepted lab test, medical scan or genetic biomarker that can definitively, diagnose or confirm this disease [6]. A diagnosis of ME/CFS is thus, typically, only rendered after "other" disorders, that present with similar symptoms, are excluded. Moreover, the varied case definitions/diagnostic criteria can add to the diagnostic uncertainty (as will be discussed later in this chapter). As a result, patients may struggle for years before receiving their diagnosis or may even be misdiagnosed and have their symptoms mistreated [6, 24]. In fact, 70% of all patients reported that they visited 4 or more doctors, and 67-77% reported that it took longer than a year, before they received their ME/CFS diagnosis. A shocking 29% reported that it took longer than 5 years before their diagnosis was rendered [42, 43]. These findings appear to support the estimated 84-91% of all ME/CFS patients remaining undiagnosed, as noted in Chapter 1 [44].

In examining the 2014 Canadian health care use data (Figure 3), one notes that individuals who experienced medically unexplained physical symptoms (MUPS) (i.e., patients experiencing ME/CFS, fibromyalgia syndrome (FMS) and multiple chemical sensitivities (MCS)), did indeed experience higher health care use. In fact, in some cases, the MUPS patients' health care use was 2-3 times higher than those of the no MUPS patients' (e.g., patients with cancer, heart disease, diabetes or asthma).

Approximately, 16% of the MUPS patients reported 10 or more visits with their general practitioner (GP) in the past year, compared to only 5% of the no MUPS patients. Additionally, approximately 53% of the MUPS patients consulted with a specialist compared to only 32% of the no MUPS, and just over one quarter (approximately, 26%) of the MUPS used a mental health service, compared to only 12% of the no MUPS. Moreover, approximately 48% of the MUPS patients required "other" medical consultations compared to only 34% of the no MUPS and approximately, 25% of the MUPS reported that their health needs were unmet verses only 11% of the no MUPS. Finally, approximately, 15% of the MUPS patients required an overnight stay at hospital, compared to only 8% of the no MUPS. Park and Gilmour [45] suggested that the higher rates of MUPS patients' health care use was likely due to their GPs referring them to specialists and other medical services to rule out "other" disorders, before rendering an "official" ME/CFS diagnosis [45].

Figure 3: Health care use and unmet needs in past year, by medically unexplained physical symptoms (MUPS) status, household population aged 25 or older, Canada, 2014

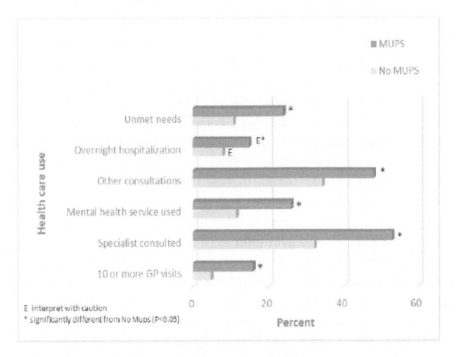

Source: Canadian Community Health Survey, 2014; cited in Park and Gilmour (2017) [45]. No MUPS includes disorders such as diabetes, cancer, heart disease and asthma.

The rendering of a ME/CFS diagnosis can be further complicated by the fact that most patients, first visit their doctors complaining of fatigue. The symptom of fatigue, however, can be the result of numerous physical and mental health conditions. Clinicians are therefore, "challenged to integrate the subjective and objective evidence that can help identify the neurologic, malignant, infectious, inflammatory, cardiopulmonary, metabolic, endocrinologic, physical deconditioning, pharmacologic, or mental health factors that may underlie the presenting complaint of fatigue" [46].

As noted earlier, a diagnosis of ME/CFS is typically, only rendered after "other" disorders that present with similar symptoms are excluded. Among these disorders are the EBV, cancer, FMS, Lyme disease, lupus, multiple sclerosis, Addison's disease, AIDS and sleep apnea. They further include depression, schizophrenia, anemia, eating disorders such as anorexia nervosa and bulimia, bipolar disorder, alcohol or another substance abuse, undertreated hypothyroidism and chronic hepatitis [2, 7, 23].

After excluding these "other" medical disorders, a ME/CFS diagnosis would only be rendered if: a) the patient has a severe and disabling fatigue that lasts for 6 months or longer, b) the fatigue is not caused by over exertion and is not substantially relieved by rest, c) the fatigue has an identifiable onset (i.e., it is not lifelong) and d) the fatigue results in a substantial reduction, of 50% or more, in the patient's previous levels of stamina. The fatigue would also need to severely compromise the individuals' occupational, educational, personal and social activities. Other disease symptoms such as pain, memory problems and unrefreshing sleep would also be present [3, 47].

The varied case definitions/criteria

As mentioned earlier, the various ME/CFS case definitions/criteria may further add to the diagnostic uncertainty. Over the years, a number of case definitions/criteria have been developed to facilitate both the medical professionals in diagnosing patients and the research community in undertaking studies. The more commonly used criteria, for both clinical and research purposes, are the Fakuda/CDC (U.S. Centers for Disease and Prevention Control) Case Definition and the Canadian Consensus Criteria (CCC) [4, 48]. The British National Institute for Health and Clinical Excellence (NICE) Guidelines and the International Consensus Criteria (ICC) are also commonly used [4, 48].

The use of these different case definitions/criteria are a source of concern for many. First, they can add to the diagnostic uncertainty of the medical professionals. Secondly, they can add to the confusion of clinicians, patients and family members alike, as the information in the public domain may be inconsistent – varying according to the definition/criteria being employed. Finally, they can be a source of concern for the research community. Over the years, researchers have operationalized these different definitions in their studies. Some studies for example, operationalized the Fakuda/CDC definition while others the CCC's. Some of the studies may, therefore, have captured the more severely impaired patients' experiences while others, the less severely impaired. This practice has resulted in study comparison limitations [4, 11]. In examining Table 4, which summarizes the four case definitions/criteria, one can easily understand many of these concerns. For a full description of the case definitions/criteria, please refer to Appendix A.

Table 4: The varied ME/CFS case definitions/criteria

Symptom	Fakuda/ CDC Case Definition [59]	CCC Criteria [49]	NICE Guidelines [58]	ICC Criteria [47, 50]
Fatigue that lasts for 6 months or more	✓			
Fatigue that results in substantial reductions in activity levels	✓	✓	✓	✓
Post exertional malaise/fatigue	4 or more of the following symptoms: ✓	✓	✓	✓
Sleep dysfunction	✓	✓	2 or more of the following 5 symptoms: ✓ (i)	*Neurological impairment categories*: at least one symptom from 3 of the following 4 symptom categories ✓ (i)

Symptom	Fakuda/ CDC Case Definition [59]	CCC Criteria [49]	NICE Guidelines [58]	ICC Criteria [47, 50]
Pain: Muscle/joint pain	✓	✓	✓ (ii)	✓ (ii)
Pain: Headaches	✓	✓	✓ (iii)	✓ (ii)
Tender lymph nodes in neck or armpit	✓	✓*		
Sore throat	✓		✓ (iv)	
Cognitive dysfunction	✓	*Neurologic/ cognitive manifestation category* (2 or more manifestations such as cognitive confusion, impaired concentration, short-term memory loss, disorientation)	✓ (v)	✓ (iii)
		Autonomic, neuroendocrine or immune manifestation categories (at least 1 symptom from 2 of these 3 categories)		Inability to focus vision, sensitivity to light, muscle weakness ✓ (iv)
		i. Autonomic: e.g., orthostatic intolerance (OI)**, neurally-mediated hypotension		

Symptom	Fakuda/ CDC Case Definition [59]	CCC Criteria [49]	NICE Guidelines [58]	ICC Criteria [47, 50]
		ii. Neuroendocrine: e.g., intolerance to extremes of heat and cold***, cold extremities		
		iii. Immune manifestation: e.g., new sensitivities to food, medications and/ or chemicals****, tender lymph nodes* Note: Symptoms from at least 2 of these 3 manifestation categories must last for 6 months or longer		*Immune, gastro-intestinal and genitourinary impairments*: at least one symptom from 3 of the following 5 symptom categories
Palpitations in the absence of cardiac pathology ***			✓	
General malaise or flu like symptoms ***			✓	✓ *(i)*
Dizziness and/or nausea, abdominal pain ***			✓	✓ *(ii)*

Symptom	Fakuda/ CDC Case Definition [59]	CCC Criteria [49]	NICE Guidelines [58]	ICC Criteria [47, 50]
Genitourinary problems: e.g., urinary urgency or frequency				✓ *(iii)*
				Susceptibility to viral infections with prolonged recovery periods *(iv)*
				Sensitivities to food, medications, odors and/or chemicals**** *(v)*
				Energy production/ transportation impairments: at least 1 symptom from the following 4 categories
				i. Cardiovascular: e.g., inability to tolerate an upright position (OI)**
				ii. Respiratory: e.g., air hunger, labored breathing
				iii. Loss of thermostatic ability: e.g., subnormal body temperature
				*iv. Intolerance to temperature extremes***

More recently, in 2015, the Committee on the Diagnostic Criteria for ME/CFS, in attempting to develop evidence-based clinical diagnostic criteria for clinicians and health care professionals alike, proposed the following ME/CFS diagnostic criteria:

1. a substantial reduction or impairment in the ability to engage in pre-illness levels of occupational, educational, social or personal activities, that persists for more than 6 months and is accompanied by fatigue, which is often profound, is of a new or definite onset (i.e., not lifelong), is not the result of ongoing excessive exertion and is not substantially alleviated by rest,
2. post-exertional malaise* and
3. unrefreshing sleep.

At least one of the following manifestations is also required:

1. cognitive impairment* or
2. orthostatic intolerance (OI).
   (* The frequency and severity of symptoms should be assessed, with the diagnosis of ME/CFS questioned if patients do not have these symptoms at least half of the time with moderate, substantial or severe intensity) [51].

Generally speaking, there are other common symptoms that would accompany the extreme fatigue, post-exertional malaise, sleep dysfunction, cognitive dysfunction and OI. Among these symptoms are pain; a lack of muscle strength; immune dysregulation difficulties; difficulty maintaining an upright position, dizziness and balance problems; allergies or sensitivities to foods, odors, chemicals, medications or noise; irritable bowel syndrome symptoms such as bloating, stomach pain, constipation, diarrhea and nausea; chills and night sweats; visual disturbances such as a sensitivity to light, blurring and eye pain; and depression or mood disorders such as irritability, mood swings, anxiety and panic attacks. Patients would also commonly experience chest pain; a chronic cough; alcohol intolerance; dry eyes or mouth; earaches; irregular heartbeat; jaw pain; morning stiffness; shortness of breath; skin sensations such as tingling; and weight loss [4, 14, 24].

Coexisting medical conditions

To complicate diagnostic matters further, many ME/CFS patients experience coexisting medical conditions. In fact, 97% of patients experience at least one other medical condition and 64% experience a psychological condition. ME/CFS patients have been found, on average, to experience between 3 and 11 coexisting medical conditions. "Multiple co-morbid conditions are [thus] the rule rather than the exception" [52]. Among the coexisting medical conditions are FMS, eating disorders such as anorexia and bulimia, multiple chemical sensitivities (MCS), irritable bowel syndrome (IBS), temporomandibular joint pain (TMJ), attention deficit and hyperactivity disorder (ADHD), depression, anxiety, sleep disorders and chronic headaches, which include migraines [2, 3, 25].

FMS is a commonly found, coexisting medical disorder in ME/CFS patients. FMS is "characterized by widespread musculoskeletal pain accompanied by fatigue, sleep, memory and mood issues. Researchers believe that FMS amplifies painful sensations by affecting the way your brain processes pain signals" (https://www.mayoclinic.org/diseases-conditions/fibromyalgia/symptoms-causes). FMS frequently occurs in ME/CFS patients between the onset and the second year of ME/CFS. Some researchers believe that FMS and ME/CFS are related disorders, as they share common symptoms such as sore throats, headaches, low grade fevers, depression, prolonged fatigue and widespread muscle aches. Other researchers suggest however, that they are two separate disorders with FMS patients experiencing more pain and ME/CFS patients experiencing more fatigue. As with ME/CFS, FMS is a chronic and non-curable disease [2, 3, 14].

Temporomandibular joint pain (TMJ) is another commonly found disorder in ME/CFS patients. TMJ can cause severe pain in the jaw joint and severe spasms in the muscles that control the movement of the jaw. The cause of TMJ is believed to be due to "a combination of factors such as genetics, arthritis, stress or jaw injury" (https://www.mayoclinic.org/diseases-conditions/tmj/symptoms-causes). While it remains unclear as to why people with ME/CFS are more prone to coexisting disorders such as TMJ and FMS, there is a theory that all of these conditions fall under the umbrella of central sensitivity syndromes. The pain associated with these disorders may contribute to the development of control sensitization problems and eventually, to central sensitivity syndromes [53].

MCS are commonly observed in ME/CFS patients, as well. With MCS, chemicals such as perfumes, fabric softeners or paint, can precipitate symptoms of extreme fatigue, nausea and overall, malaise [3]. MCS, like ME/CFS, is a chronic disorder. Finally, mood disorders are very, common coexisting medical conditions. Typically, ME/CFS patients experience more depression, tension and anxiety than that of the healthy population [54, 55]. In fact, 40% of all ME/CFS patients experience some level of depression, anxiety or irritability [12]. Some researchers suggest that the coexistence of the mood disorders may be the result of clinical manifestations of shared inflammatory pathways [56] while, other researchers suggest that the mood disorders are comorbid or secondary, to the ME/CFS disease state. That is to say, the ME/CFS disease state precedes or precipitates the psychological and social dysfunction [39, 57]. The stress of living with the numerous and unexplained symptoms, and their debilitating effects on patients' lives, may be the cause of these mood disorders [45].

Finally, there has been some debate as to whether the coexisting medical disorders may actually be the cause of ME/CFS. Some researchers posit that some of the coexisting medical disorders may precipitate the onset of ME/CFS by years and then, become associated with it later-on [14, 50]. I can certainly relate to this hypothesis, as I experienced a number of the above noted coexisting medical disorders, prior to my ME/CFS diagnosis. In my early 20s for example, I developed an eating disorder, in my 30s I developed TMJ and irritable bowel syndrome (IBS), and in my 40s, I experienced chronic migraines. The TMJ, IBS and migraines have continued throughout my journey with ME/CFS. As with many other patients, my journey with ME/CFS has also resulted in a diagnosis of FMS.

The Canadian data on the comorbidity of ME/CFS, FMS and MCS, as depicted in Table 5, certainly confirm much of the above noted discussions. Just over half (50.7%) of all MUPS patients, which in some instances only includes ME/CFS and MCS, reported having three or more chronic, physical conditions compared, to only 12.9% of the no MUPS patients (e.g., patients with cancer, heart disease, asthma or diabetes). Furthermore, almost a quarter (22.7%) of the MUPS patients reported some form of accompanying mental disorder (i.e., depression, general anxiety or a mood disorder), compared to only 7.6% of the no MUPS patients. Of the mental disorders reported by the MUPS patients, the mood or anxiety disorders were the highest reported at 34.7%, compared to only 10.3% of the no MUPS patients.

In examining the ME/CFS patients' experiences specifically, 64.7% reported the prevalence of 3 or more chronic, physical conditions. This figure is higher than that of the MCS (40.6%), FMS (63.5%) and no MUPS patient (12.9%) groups. Moreover, the ME/CFS patients reported the highest rates of major depressive disorder (26.2%), general anxiety disorder (18.7%), mood or anxiety disorder (54.3%) and any mental disorder (34.7%). In many cases, the ME/CFS figures were twice as high as those of the MCS and more than 4-6 times higher than the no MUPS. On the basis of this data, ME/CFS patients experience higher incidences of comorbid physical and mental conditions, than any of the other patient groups.

Table 5: Prevalence of physical and mental comorbidity for ME/CFS, MCS and Fibromyalgia, household population aged 25 and older, 2012 and 2014

Household population by disorder and physical and mental condition	Any MUPS*	Chronic Fatigue Syndrome (ME/CFS)	Multiple Chemical Sensitivity (MCS)	Fibromyalgia (FMS)	No MUPS **
A) Chronic physical conditions					
None	9.8	6.0	12.5	5.7	45.7
One	18.4	12.4	24.7	10.9	26.5
Two	21.1	16.9	22.2	19.9	14.9
3 or more	50.7	64.7	40.6	63.5	12.9

So, what is ME/CFS and how does it manifest itself?

Household population by disorder and physical and mental condition	Any MUPS*	Chronic Fatigue Syndrome (ME/CFS)	Multiple Chemical Sensitivity (MCS)	Fibromyalgia (FMS)	No MUPS **
B) Mental disorders					
Major depressive episode	15.5*	26.2	12.6	N/A	3.8**
General anxiety disorder	10.7*	18.7	8.3	N/A	2.2**
Mood or anxiety disorder	34.7*	54.3	27.2	40.9***	10.3**
Any mental disorder	22.7*	34.7	18.8	N/A	7.6**
Comorbidity with ME/CFS ***		-	15	30	
Comorbidity with FMS***		23	13	-	
Comorbidity with MCS***		9	-	10	

Notes: Any MUPS: * includes only ME/CFS and MCS; ** No MUPS: excludes only ME/CFS and MCS; No MUPS includes disorders such as diabetes, cancer, heart disease and asthma. *** based on data from 2014 Canadian Community Health Survey.

Sources: 2012 Canadian Community Health Survey–Mental Health and 2014 Canadian Community Health Survey, cited in Park and Gilmour (2017) [45].

The comorbidity of FMS and MCS among ME/CFS patients is also quite substantial. Thirty percent of all ME/CFS patients for example, reported also suffering from FMS and 15% from MCS. Twenty three percent of FMS patients, on the other hand, suffered from ME/CFS and 13% from MCS while, 9% of MCS patients suffered from ME/CFS and 10% from FMS [45]. On the basis of this data, ME/CFS patients experience higher incidences of comorbid FMS and MCS medical conditions.

When one takes into consideration the fact that 2% of all Canadians report a diagnosis of fibromyalgia, 2.7% MCS and 1.6% ME/CFS [45], we are talking about 6.3% of the Canadian population living with one of these

55

three disorders. In other words, approximately 1.6 million Canadians suffer from one of these three chronic, invisible and disabling diseases. Given that these three disorders frequently co-exist, patients may not only suffer from the varied symptoms of one of these three "primary" disorders but, they may also suffer from the symptoms of the other two conditions, as well. The challenges of living with the numerous and debilitating symptoms of ME/CFS, MCS or FMS alone, can be difficult for patients. Living with the symptoms of all three disorders, acting in tandem, can make the ME/CFS disease state even more challenging, devastating and burdensome. These three disorders, all acting in tandem, can exact a very heavy toll on the patients' lifestyle, employment, financial independence and overall sense of well-being,

Grading the severity of ME/CFS

As previously mentioned, in the months following my ME/CFS diagnosis, I had difficulty understanding why some individuals reportedly returned to health within six months of their disease onset while, I remained bedridden for almost the entire first year. It was not until I came upon the information pertaining to the grading of ME/CFS that I began to understand some of the reasons for these differences. The ME/CFS disease spectrum is fairly, broad and ranges from a mild to a more moderate, severe or very severe case. The severity of the patients' disease state can make all the difference in their ME/CFS experiences and recovery time.

According to the NICE guidelines [58], the severity of ME/CFS ranges from mild to moderate and severe/very severe. A mild case would include individuals who are mobile, can care for themselves and can undertake light, domestic tasks without difficulty. Most of these individuals would still be working. However, in order for these individuals to remain at work, they would likely have ceased all leisure and social pursuits and would need to take days off, in order to continue with their work life. Most of these individuals would also need to use the weekends to cope with their upcoming work week. A moderate case would involve a reduced mobility and a restriction in all daily activities. Peaks and troughs of ability would occur, depending on the degree of the patients' symptoms. These individuals would usually have stopped work and would require rest periods including, sleeping in the afternoon for one or two hours a day. Sleep quality at night would also be generally poor and disturbed. Finally, a severe/very severe case would include individuals who can carry out only minimal daily tasks such as face washing and teeth cleaning or, who are unable to mobilize and do any tasks for themselves. These individuals would also have severe cognitive difficulties, may be wheelchair dependent for mobility and would be unable to leave the house, except on rare occasions, followed by severe and prolonged after-effects from their efforts. Additionally, these patients would be extremely sensitive to light, unable to tolerate noise and in bed most of the time.

The ICC, on the other hand, grades the severity of this disease a little differently. The ICC's grading ranges from mild to moderate, severe and very severe. Under the ICC criteria, symptom severity must result in a significant reduction in the patients' premorbid activity levels. A mild case of ME/CFS would see an approximate 50% reduction in the patients' pre-illness activity level, a moderate would see the patient mostly housebound, a severe mostly bedridden and a very severe, totally bedridden and requiring help with basic functions. The ICC further notes that there may be marked fluctuations in the symptom severity from day-to-day and hour-to-hour [47, 50]. On the basis of these two grading systems, the disease spectrum is fairly broad, with patients' experiences varying according to the severity of their disease state. Some patients may therefore, return relatively quickly to their premorbid health levels while, other patients, as will be discussed in Chapter 5, may struggle for years with ME/CFS [12].

In summation, my journey through the research literature outlined in this chapter has helped me to understand what ME/CFS is, its risk factors and its possible causes. It has also helped me to understand why there may be misconceptions and judgements from "others" about this disease and the individuals who struggle with it – ME/CFS is a complex, invisible disorder for which there is no known underlying medical condition, no known cause and no means of confirming its diagnosis. Moreover, the use of the varied case definitions/criteria only add to the misunderstandings and confusion surrounding this disease. By delving into the definitions/criteria and the grading of the disease, I now better understand my numerous and varied symptoms, and my more severe disease experiences. I also better appreciate that my experiences in receiving a ME/CFS diagnosis were very similar to those of other patients' – it takes time as other diseases, which present with similar symptoms, must first be ruled out through medical tests and consultations with various medical specialists. My experiences with the coexisting medical conditions were also validated and thankfully, I now understand that I am not becoming a "mean dragon lady" but am simply living with a chronic and debilitating disease. My mood disorders, while I continue to struggle with them and wish that they were not a part of my life, are coexisting conditions and are a natural consequence of the ME/CFS disease state. I, finally, have some goal posts or roadmap by which to understand and assess my ME/CFS experiences, and now comprehend that I am living with a complex disorder of unknown cause, numerous, varied and relentless symptoms, coexisting medical disorders that add to the complexity of the disease state and a broad spectrum of symptom severity. Overall, these research findings have provided me with a level of knowledge that I very much needed to move forward. In many respects, this literature has been comforting and liberating for me.

Now that we have an appreciation of ME/CFS in more general terms and some of its complexities, let's dig a little deeper. Chapter 4 will examine the five core ME/CFS symptom categories and the extent to which they can challenge and debilitate patients' lives. As we shall discover, this disease, while not apparent to an onlooker, is not "all in the patient's head". In fact, patients' experiences with this devastating, complex, multi-system disease have been objectively measured, through both quantitative and qualitative means.

Chapter 4

ME/CFS IS NOT
"ALL IN THE PATIENT'S HEAD"

*If you want others to be happy, practice compassion. If you want
to be happy practice compassion*

~ *Dalai Lama*

*When we meet real tragedy in life, we can react in two ways –
either by losing hope and falling into self-destructive habits, or by
using the challenge to find our inner strength*

~ *Dalai Lama*

When I was first diagnosed with ME/CFS, I thought that I would recover fairly, quickly. Afterall, ME/CFS sounded like a disease that, with a lot of sleep and rest, would see me once again enjoying my life. As time passed however, I discovered that no amount of sleep or rest was restorative. Moreover, this disease was so severe that I could barely move or function, and every movement or activity, no matter how insignificant, would exacerbate my many symptoms and send me scurrying back to bed for endless hours of sleep and bedrest. I was so physically, cognitively and spiritually challenged that I struggled to meet the simplest of my life's demands. In many respects, I was no longer able to do, think or be the person who I most wanted to be. I felt lost, alone, bewildered and in despair. I could not believe that this rather benign sounding, invisible disease could be so crippling, so all life consuming.

It was not until I came upon the core, ME/CFS symptom categories that I began to more deeply appreciate that I was suffering from a devastating, complex, multi-system disease. While Chapter 3 explored ME/CFS in more general terms, this chapter will explore this chronic, invisible, multi-system disease and its devastating impacts on patients' lives.

Living with ME/CFS: While ME/CFS may be invisible to others, it is most definitely not "all in the patient's head"

Oft times in this more evidence-based world, if something cannot be seen, measured or proven, its reality is brought into question. ME/CFS is certainly a case in point. As a chronic and invisible disease, ME/CFS is not obvious to an onlooker. Moreover, there is no known cause, no known underlying medical condition and no known lab test or medical scan that can confirm or diagnose it [1, 2]. ME/CFS can, therefore, be overlooked, downplayed, misunderstood and judged by "others" [3]. It can also leave "others" questioning if the disease is real or whether it is "all in the patient's head". These misconceptions, misunderstandings and judgements are very unfortunate, as patients are often left to quietly struggle alone, both with the disease itself and "others'" misconceptions about it.

Fortunately, the ME/CFS research literature has quantified and qualified patients' disease experiences. The research evidence is quite compelling, ME/CFS is real! In fact, ME/CFS is regarded as a clinical disorder of biochemical and physiological abnormalities. These biochemical and physiological abnormalities affect multiple body systems [4, 5] and cause "dysfunction [in the patients'] neurological, immune, endocrine and energy/metabolism systems" [6].

The research has identified nine symptom categories that speak to this multi-system disease and the dysfunction that it can cause. The five core symptom categories or, the symptoms that are most universally present and severe in patients' disease experiences, are impaired day-to-day functioning due to the debilitating fatigue, post exertional malaise (PEM), sleep related disorders, cognitive impairments and orthostatic intolerance (OI) [6, 7]. The four secondary symptom categories relate to pain, infection, immune impairment and neuroendocrine manifestations. These latter symptom categories will not be explored in this book as they are typically, the less frequent and severe in patients' ME/CFS experiences [6]. It should be noted however, that symptoms from each of these nine symptom categories can present themselves, to varying degrees, in the patients' disease experience. The possible accumulation of symptoms from each of these nine symptom categories, only adds to the complexity of living with this disease and "contributes significantly to the burden imposed … by this illness" [8]. It will also be recalled that patients' disease experiences will vary according to the number, type, severity and duration of their symptoms [8]. Figure 4 provides a graphic depiction of the possible disease state, when all nine symptom categories are present in the patient's disease experience while, Figure 5 presents the case of this multi-system disease.

**Figure 4: A depiction of the core and secondary
ME/CFS symptom categories**

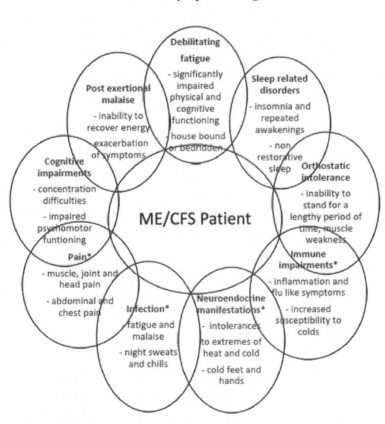

* Secondary ME/CFS symptom categories. **Sources:** Institute of Medicine (2015) [5] and ME/CFS case definitions/criteria as outlined in Appendix A.

Impaired day-to-day functioning due to the debilitating fatigue

Let's face it, many individuals in today's society are fatigued, to varying degrees, by the daily demands of their lives. We live in a society of incessant demands, quick turnarounds and little downtime. Fatigue can be a natural consequence of this lifestyle. The fatigue associated with ME/CFS however, is described as "more intense and qualitatively different" than that of normal fatigue and tiredness [9]. It represents a "pathophysiological exhaustion" [10] that leaves an estimated 25% of all patients bedridden, socially isolated and dependent on others for their daily care [11]. Moreover, the fatigue is not the result of excessive exertion, is not life-long (i.e., it has an identifiable start) and is not alleviated by rest [12]. The fatigue is also accompanied by numerous other symptoms such as "weakness, heaviness, general malaise, light headedness and sleepiness that can be overwhelming" [13]. This fatigue can severely reduce the individuals' ability to function and fully participate in their physical and mental lives [11, 14], and often results in patients having great difficulty staying on top of their work, home, family and social responsibilities [14, 15].

The fatigue associated with ME/CFS has been further described as "more profound, more devastating and longer lasting than that observed in patients with other fatiguing disorders" [16]. In fact, the fatigue levels associated with ME/CFS are believed to be similar to those of patients undergoing chemotherapy, and suffering from HIV (until about two weeks before death), cancer, multiple sclerosis, Lyme disease or congestive heart failure [16, 17].

The fatigue can be triggered in a variety of ways. Among these are: a) physical exertion [18], b) cognitive exertion [19], c) emotional distress [20], d) decreased sleep quantity and quality [21], e) an infection [22] and e) standing or sitting up for an extended period of time [22]. Once the fatigue is triggered, patients can be rendered highly, functionally impaired [23, 24], can experience an exacerbation of many other symptoms and are unable to pursue any level of subsequent activity [25]. In fact, many patients have great difficulty recovering their energy capacity, following even the slightest of physical, cognitive and emotional activity [18]. Furthermore, the fatigue can leave patients significantly, less active throughout their day

[26], and can severely impair their mobility and ability to function in their daily lives [24].

Figure 5: The case of a multi-system disease: Examples of the numerous and varied ME/CFS symptoms and their associated body systems

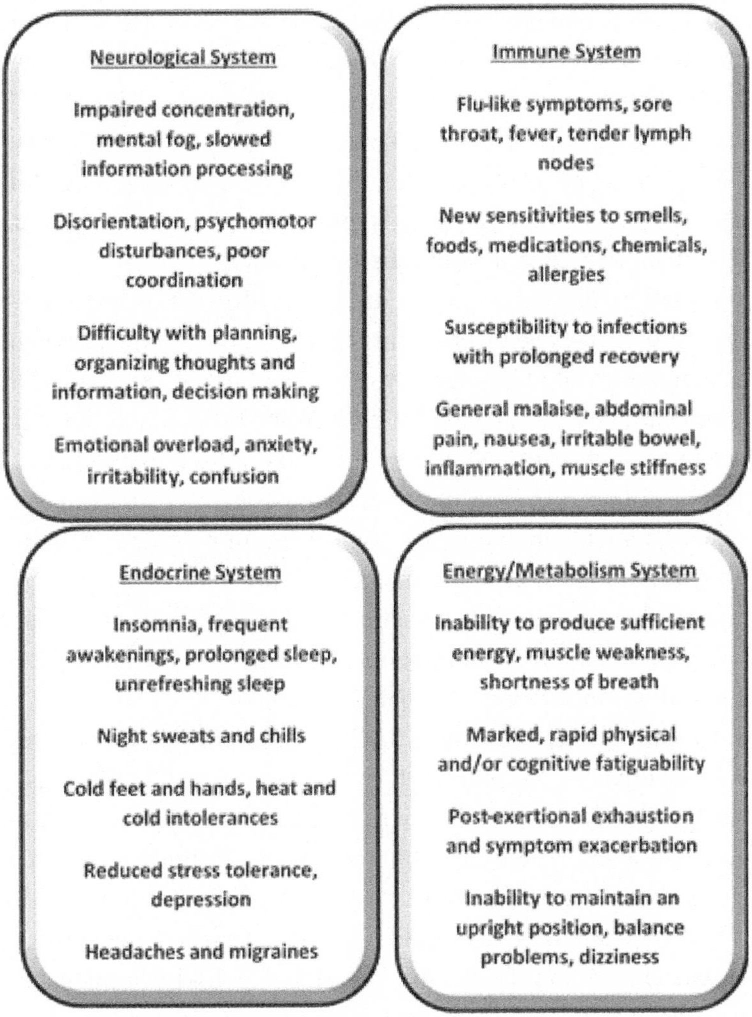

Neurological System

Impaired concentration, mental fog, slowed information processing

Disorientation, psychomotor disturbances, poor coordination

Difficulty with planning, organizing thoughts and information, decision making

Emotional overload, anxiety, irritability, confusion

Immune System

Flu-like symptoms, sore throat, fever, tender lymph nodes

New sensitivities to smells, foods, medications, chemicals, allergies

Susceptibility to infections with prolonged recovery

General malaise, abdominal pain, nausea, irritable bowel, inflammation, muscle stiffness

Endocrine System

Insomnia, frequent awakenings, prolonged sleep, unrefreshing sleep

Night sweats and chills

Cold feet and hands, heat and cold intolerances

Reduced stress tolerance, depression

Headaches and migraines

Energy/Metabolism System

Inability to produce sufficient energy, muscle weakness, shortness of breath

Marked, rapid physical and/or cognitive fatiguability

Post-exertional exhaustion and symptom exacerbation

Inability to maintain an upright position, balance problems, dizziness

Source: Institute of Medicine (2015) [4], research cited in Chapters 3 and 4, and information contained in the case definitions/criteria, as outlined in Appendix A.

The impact of the fatigue can be quite profound. In fact, when compared to individuals suffering from other chronic and fatiguing disorders, ME/CFS patients experienced significantly, more impairment in their physical and cognitive functions, as measured by "vitality" scores. Patients with congestive heart failure for example, were found to have a vitality score of 29, those with major depression a score of 40 and those with chronic hepatitis a score of 48. Patients with fibromyalgia and rheumatoid arthritis, on the other hand, had vitality scores between 39-40 and 43-52 respectively, while the healthy controls scored between 50-60 points. The ME/CFS patients' scores, however, were in the range of 15-25 points, the lowest of all scores [27]. On the basis of this data, the fatigue associated with ME/CFS has a more profound effect on patients' physical and cognitive functioning, than that of the other chronic and fatiguing diseases.

In summation, the fatigue associated with ME/CFS is anything but an ordinary fatigue. In fact, it represents a "pathophysiological exhaustion" [10] that is not alleviated by sleep or rest. The fatigue can be so debilitating that an estimated 25% of all patients are bedridden and dependent on others for their daily care. Moreover, once the fatigue is triggered, many of the patients' other ME/CFS symptoms are intensified. In most cases, the fatigue causes patients to experience significant impairment in their physical and cognitive functions and renders them unable to fully participate in their personal, family, occupational and social lives. The fatigue associated with ME/CFS, which has been quantified and qualified, can be extremely debilitating, life limiting and life changing.

I can personally attest to the ME/CFS fatigue levels being similar, to those of individuals experiencing other fatiguing disorders, such as cancer or chemotherapy. When my mom was first diagnosed with cancer and undergoing chemotherapy, I noticed that she went from a very, high energy person to one who was extremely fatigued throughout the day. Mom required sleep in the afternoon, went to bed very, early in the evening and got up much later in the morning. She was sleeping 13-14 hours each night. These new sleep requirements were highly, unusual for my mom. During this period, mom and I shared very, similar energy levels, lifestyle and sleep requirements. Following mom's surgery and chemotherapy treatments, she returned to her former high energy levels while I continued, to struggle with mine.

Along similar lines, I recall an experience that I had with my dad during his short battle with cancer. My dad, like me, believed that if we set our mind to something, we can accomplish it on the basis of our will power, intention and action. When my dad first saw me struggling with high levels of fatigue, he would sometimes comment "Deb, tell yourself you can do it – you can overcome the tiredness". Sadly, about a month before my dad's passing, I recall him saying "Deb, I never thought that anyone could be this tired. I am sorry that I judged your level of fatigue. I think I understand now". God bless him for sharing that powerful, validating moment with me, and for being such a loving father and friend.

As I mentioned in Chapter 2, of all my physical challenges, fatigue was by far the most challenging. For the first year following my diagnosis, for all intents and purposes, I was bedridden, requiring 18-20 hours of sleep each day. Had I not experienced such profound levels of fatigue I would never have believed them to be humanly possible. The deep, physical exhaustion permeated everything that I did, making my life one huge struggle. So many times, I just wanted to cry, I had such difficulty meeting the most modest of my life's demands. The fatigue was overwhelming, debilitating and devastating to the life that I once lived and loved.

Post exertional malaise (PEM)

Post exertional malaise (PEM) is another core ME/CFS symptom category. PEM is defined as "the worsening of a patient's symptoms and functions after exposure to physical or cognitive [or emotional] stressors that were normally tolerated before disease onset" [28]. Among these stressors are physical trauma, infection, decreased sleep quantity and quality [22] and acute exercise [29]. PEM can immediately follow a period of physical, cognitive or emotional exertion or it can be delayed from 1 to 7 days, following the exertion experience [4, 22]. The individuals' period of recovery, subsequent to even the briefest of exertion experience, can be inordinately long, lasting for hours, days, weeks or even months [22, 30, 31]. A simple exertion experience such as talking on the telephone [32] or watching television can trigger PEM [22].

As with the fatigue, PEM can exacerbate many of the patients' other symptoms. Among these symptoms are a sore throat, nausea, tender lymph nodes [33], headaches, muscle and joint pain [34], impaired thinking processes, short-term memory loss, and a reduced ability to focus and sustain attention [35]. PEM can also exacerbate the symptoms of fatigue, weakness/instability, vertigo and sensitivity to noise [33] as well as, hypersomnia and difficulties in falling or staying asleep [36, 37]. PEM can further delay patients' muscle function recovery [38], increase depression or mood disturbances such as anxiety and irritability [19, 39], and exacerbate patients' pain levels [20, 36]. Finally, PEM can impair patients' cognitive performance and brain function, and has detrimental neurophysiological effects [29].

The repercussions of PEM on patients' lives are quite extensive. ME/CFS patients typically, experience PEM 69-100% of the time [40, 41, 42]. In comparison, healthy controls tend to experience PEM only 4-8% of the time [43, 44]. Studies further show that 86% of patients experienced physical tiredness after minimal physical exercise compared to only 7% of the healthy controls while, 85% of patients reported being drained after a mild activity verses only 2% of the healthy controls. Moreover, 83% of patients reported being sore after non-strenuous activity verses 4%, and 69% of patients reported cognitive tiredness after the slightest effort verses only 4% [27]. Finally, the more physically or cognitively active patients were, the greater the exacerbation of their symptoms and activity restrictions in the subsequent days [25].

In a more recent study, 90% of the ME/CFS patients experienced PEM following a physical, cognitive or emotional exertion experience. Of the symptoms that were most, commonly exacerbated by those experiences were fatigue, cognitive difficulties, sleep disturbances, headaches, muscle pain and flu-like symptoms, respectively. Gastrointestinal, orthostatic, mood-related and neurologic symptoms were also commonly exacerbated. Furthermore, 84% of the patients endured PEM for a period of 24 hours or more while, 11% experienced a post-trigger delay of, at least, 24 hours before the onset of their symptoms [45].

As a result of PEM, many patients experience increased and prolonged levels of fatigue, and have great difficulty recovering their energy levels following an exertion experience [37, 38]. In studying patients' recovery times, or their ability to return to their prior levels of functioning following an exertion experience, ME/CFS patients were found to need significantly, longer recovery times than the healthy controls. One study for example, found that 100% of the healthy controls experienced a full, physical recovery within a 24-48-hour period following an exertion experience while, only 31% of the ME/CFS patients were able to do so. Moreover, 60% of the ME/CFS patients continued to experience varied symptoms, such as debilitating fatigue, pain, muscle fatigue and a lack of endurance, for a week following the exertion experience [18]. Significant cognitive impairments are also commonly found in patients post exertion [35, 46, 47, 48]. In one study, patients required an average of 57 hours to return to their pretest mental energy levels, compared to only a 7-hour recovery period for the healthy controls [49]. Quite a stark contrast!

Interestingly, some immune biomarkers have been identified in patients, following a physical exertion experience [30, 50, 51, 52, 53]. Among these biomarkers are significantly reduced miRNAs. These miRNAs are believed to suppress certain translation processes involved in the cellular development and immune functions of patients [54]. In addition, increases in IgAs/IGM responses, associated with inflammation and cell mediated immune activation, have also been identified in patients [39, 47] as well as, plasma interleukin (IL-I), tumor necrosis (TNFa) and neopterin – all disease fighting cells [55]. These genetic biomarkers may eventually lead to a better understanding of the pathophysiology of ME/CFS, as they appear to affect the patients' immune functions and the severity of their symptoms including, their mood disorders (e.g., sadness and irritability) [2, 51]. Finally, the severity and duration of the patients' PEM symptoms are believed to be predictors of poorer patient outcomes and may thus, be important indicators of patients' prognoses [56].

In summation, PEM is associated with the worsening of patients' symptoms and functions, following exposure to the slightest of physical, cognitive or emotional exertion. PEM can require an inordinately, long recovery time, lasting anywhere from hours, days, weeks or even months, following even the most modest of activities. The effects of PEM on patients' lives are quite extensive, ranging from extreme fatigue to cognitive difficulties, muscle and joint pain, sleep dysfunction and mood disorders. The effects of PEM, when compared to those of the healthy controls, are significantly more restrictive on ME/CFS patients. The immune biomarkers that have been identified in patients following an exertion experience may, in time, lead to a better understanding of the pathophysiology of ME/CFS. PEM, like the effects of the debilitating fatigue, can profoundly impact the patients' ability to function and participate in their personal, family, work and social lives.

I too struggled with PEM on my ME/CFS journey. Any amount of physical, cognitive or emotional exertion, no matter how inconsequential, left me physically, cognitively and spiritually exhausted – unable to function and participate in my life. PEM really intensified my numerous symptoms including fatigue, overall malaise, pain, headaches, cognitive exhaustion, sleep dysfunction and mood disorders. Any attempt at trying to have some semblance of a normal life, like having family or close friends over for a short visit or chatting on the telephone, were met with PEM. There was no escaping PEM nor its impact on my life! In many respects, PEM made my already limited life even more limited, making an already difficult situation, even more difficult. PEM has been very, concerning and debilitating for me. The struggles and deep despair that accompanied PEM, could be crushing.

PEM has made the writing of this book very, challenging. If I was able to write for a couple of hours a day, for two consecutive days, I was left extremely physically, cognitively and spiritually fatigued, required endless hours of sleep and bedrest, and experienced migraines, weakness, dizziness, irritability, frustration and sadness. I was frequently unable to return to my writing for weeks or months at a time. Furthermore, when engaged in the act of writing itself, I experienced cognitive difficulties such as an inability to sustain my attention, to clearly and concisely put forward my ideas, to have my ideas flow in a logical manner and to remember what I had just written. I, consequently, often thought about walking away from this book – the physical, cognitive and spiritual consequences seemed too high a price to pay. Writing, a once joyful, easy and creative process had become such a taxing, frustrating and demeaning endeavor. But the writing of this book was cathartic and gave me a sense of purpose. It kept me moving forward, something that I very much needed in my life.

Sleep related disorders

The sleep related disorders that ME/CFS patients experience can be equally challenging. These disorders include insomnia, frequent or sustained awakenings throughout the night, and nonrestorative or unrefreshing sleep [22, 57]. The sleep disorders also tend to be chronic, with the insomnia and frequent or sustained awakenings often occurring when patients are overly exhausted [58, 59]. Only a small percentage of patients fail to report some type of sleep disorder, with most patients reporting sleep related difficulties at least half of the time [27]. The sleep manifestations, like the debilitating fatigue and PEM, can result in substantial reductions in the patients' functions and activity levels including, their work productivity [4].

In examining patients' sleep related experiences, relative to those of the healthy controls, studies show that 92% of ME/CFS patients experienced unrefreshing sleep compared to only 16% of the healthy controls while, 68% of the patients had problems falling asleep verses only 22% of the healthy controls. Moreover, 65% of patients needed to nap daily verses 10%, 58% had problems staying asleep verses 21%, 47% woke up very early in the morning verses 15% and finally, 14% either slept all day or were awake all-night verses only 4% [27]. ME/CFS patients also reported significantly, more sleepiness and fatigue throughout their day than the healthy controls [60]. In addition, many patients reported high levels of microarousal during the night and spent significantly, more time awake after sleep onset [61, 62, 63]. Finally, patients' sleep patterns changed over time with many patients complaining of hypersomnia in the first few months of their illness but, as the disease progressed, they had trouble remaining asleep [64].

The research suggests that the sleep related disorders may be due to the patients' higher levels of cortisol and heart rate variability (HRV). The higher cortisol levels, found in some patients, may be responsible for the delay in their ability to fall asleep and have a normal and refreshing night's sleep. These higher levels of cortisol may be responsible for stimulating the patients' sleep arousal [65]. In terms of HRV, ME/CFS patients have been found to be 7 times more likely, than the healthy controls, to experience repeated awakenings throughout the night as well as, a poorer quality of sleep [66]. Reductions in some patients' vagal HRV are believed to be the cause of these repeated awakenings and the pervasive state of nocturnal hypervigilance [66] (Note: the vagal nerve is responsible for the regulation of several body organs at rest and results in various effects including, heart rate reduction, glandular activity in the heart, lungs and digestive tract, and immune system regulation) (https://en.wikipedia.org/wiki/Vagal_tone). Finally, a beat-to-beat HRV, observed during some ME/CFS patients' non-rapid eye movement (REM) sleep, may explain some of the disruptive sleep patterns [67].

Many ME/CFS patients undergo sleep studies to determine if their sleep disorders are "primary" sleep disorders and thus, treatable. Typically, a primary sleep disorder would rule out a diagnosis of ME/CFS. However, primary sleep disorders are more commonly being observed in ME/CFS patients. In fact, the prevalence of "primary" sleep disorders in ME/CFS patients range from 19-69% [69, 70] and include, restless leg syndrome (1-4%), periodic limb movement disorder (4-25%), sleep apnea (13-65%) and narcolepsy (5-7%) [68, 69, 71]. Moreover, 21.1% of patients were found to experience a primary, comorbid sleep disorder, that did not invalidate their ME/CFS diagnosis [72]. Primary sleep disorders such as sleep apnea and narcolepsy are increasingly, being regarded as comorbid ME/CFS conditions (i.e., they are brought on by the ME/CFS disease state itself) [73, 74] and are, therefore, no longer being viewed as exclusionary criteria for a ME/CFS diagnosis [75]. According to the Institute of Medicine, the "diagnosis of a primary sleep disorder does not rule out a diagnosis of ME/CFS" [76].

The research literature further notes that while effective treatments do exist to address primary sleep disorders, there is little evidence to suggest that these treatments are effective in addressing ME/CFS patients' sleep related symptoms. A continuous positive airway pressure (CPAP) system for example, is a common treatment for sleep apnea. To date however, reports of a CPAP system improving ME/CFS patients' sleep related symptoms have been limited [77]. Furthermore, prescribed medications, while helpful in addressing some ME/CFS patients' sleep related disorders, can worsen other patients' sleep concerns [78, 79]. Sleep treatments and medications may not, therefore, be appropriate in addressing all ME/CFS patients' sleep related disorders [78, 79].

In summation, the ME/CFS sleep related disorders include insomnia, frequent or sustained awakenings throughout the night and nonrestorative sleep. These disorders also tend to be chronic with most patients experiencing sleep related difficulties at least 50% of the time. Relative to the healthy controls, ME/CFS patients report significantly, higher levels of sleep related problems. According to the research, these sleep related challenges may be related to biochemical and physiological abnormalities, such as higher levels of cortisol and HRV. Finally, the sleep related disorders can significantly impair the patients' functioning and ability to live their daily lives.

I too have experienced sleep related disorders on my ME/CFS journey. As mentioned previously, for almost the entire first year following my diagnosis, I slept incessantly. Sleep consumed my life! As time passed, as with many other patients' experiences, I was either unable to fall asleep for hours on end or I would wake up incessantly throughout the entire night. I felt like I was awakening every 15 to 20 minutes. It was exhausting! To this day, I continue to struggle with sleep related concerns. I frequently wake up feeling unrefreshed regardless of the amount of sleep that I get, and if I am overly tired, I can either not fall asleep or cannot remain asleep. Some nights, I am so tired when I go to bed that I want to cry and yet, I cannot fall asleep. The levels of fatigue, malaise and dysfunction that can result from these sleep related disorders are very, challenging. In many respects, they compound my existing levels of fatigue and further reduce my ability to function in my life.

Part of my ME/CFS journey involved my participation in sleep studies as well, to determine if my sleep concerns were "primary" sleep related disorders and treatable. My first two sleep studies were normal. My third and more in-depth study however, revealed that I had an upper airway disorder. According to the sleep specialist, this disorder was impairing my breathing and causing me to be in a more awakened state throughout the night. The specialist believed that this disorder was due to a restricted nasal passage, caused by a broken nose that I had sustained in childhood. The doctor suggested that I try a CPAP system but recommended a septoplasty. He stated that the septoplasty would permanently address my upper airway disorder. After consulting with my general practitioner (my primary doctor) and a surgeon, I opted for the surgery. Subsequent to the surgery, while I continue to have nights where I can either not fall asleep or awake countless times throughout the night, I do feel that on a good night, I am getting a deeper and more restful night's sleep. I am now able for example, to enter the dream state – a sign that I am entering a deeper and more restorative sleep phase. I am certainly, not advocating surgery for individuals in similar situations, I am simply stating that the surgery was helpful to me.

Cognitive impairments

The cognitive impairments associated with ME/CFS are numerous and varied and they too, can greatly impact the patients' day-to-day functioning. These impairments include overall mental fatigue, short term memory problems, an impaired ability to sustain attention and difficulty remembering something that was just read [80, 81]. They additionally include, moderate to large impairments in simple and complex information processing speed, in working memory over a sustained period of time [80, 81], and in encoding and processing information [82]. A hypersensitivity to sensory stimulation such as noise, bright lights, odors and temperature extremes [83] as well as, impairments in executive attention and multitasking (most particularly, when confronted with distractions such as noise or a fast-paced environment) are also common [84]. Finally, patients can experience impaired psychomotor functioning (e.g., slowed reaction and movement times) [85, 86], and impaired psychomotor disturbances (e.g., muscle weakness, poor muscle coordination and a loss of balance) [87]. The cognitive manifestations are believed to be more impactful on the patients' functional status and well-being than those of other chronic diseases [89]. In fact, the cognitive impairments associated with ME/CFS are "responsible for the disability that results in (the patients') loss of employment and loss of functional capacity in social environments" [90].

When comparing the effects of the cognitive impairments on the patients' functional status, relative to those of the healthy controls, studies have found that 80% of ME/CFS patients experienced memory related problems compared to only 7% of the healthy controls. Moreover, 73% of patients had difficulty expressing their thoughts verses 2%, and 69% had difficulty paying attention verses 7%. Furthermore, 68% of patients experienced issues with absent mindedness verses only 5%, 66% experienced a slowed thought process verses 2%, and 55% had difficulty understanding what was said verses 2% [27]. Finally, 75.5% of patients reported difficulties with word retrieval [91]. The impacts of the cognitive manifestations on patients' day-to-day living are clearly, quite substantial.

The cognitive impairments that patients experience may actually, be associated with neurological changes, changes that are objectively different from those of the healthy controls. These neurological changes include significantly lower cerebral blood flow, which may play a role in the patients' cognitive impairments and activity restrictions [92], and changes in the patients' neural circuitry (i.e., basal ganglia). These neural circuitry changes may be responsible for the impaired or reduced motor speeds that patients experience [93], as the basal ganglia is responsible for motor control as well as, motor learning and executive functions (https://www.ncbi.nlm.nih.gov/pmc/articles/PMC3543080). These neurological changes further include reduced brain activity in regions of the brain associated with working memory [94] and an increased activation in neural resources. ME/CFS patients typically, require more neural resources than the healthy controls, to achieve the same level of behavioral performance [95, 96].

Among the other neurological changes that have been observed in patients are a reduced volume of brain grey matter. On average, an 8% reduction of grey brain tissue was identified in patients [97]. Yet, other studies have observed, at fatigue onset, a reduced volume of both midbrain white and grey brain matter. This finding is believed to be consistent with an insult to the midbrain, which can lead to the distorted processing of peripheral signals including, autonomic pathway activation (i.e., the means whereby the central nervous system (CNS) sends commands to the body) and psychomotor functioning [98, 99]. Finally, an activated or inflamed microglia was found in the amygdala, thalamus and midbrain of some patients. This neuroinflammation may be responsible for some of the cognitive impairments associated with ME/CFS, such as attention deficits [100]. The microglia are a type of neuroglia (i.e., glial cell) located throughout the brain and spinal cord and account for 10–15% of all cells found within the brain. These cells act as the first and main form of active immune defense in the central nervous system (CNS) and are key cells in overall, brain maintenance (https://en.wikipedia.org/wiki/Microglia).

In summary, the cognitive impairments associated with ME/CFS are numerous and include mental fatigue, slowed information processing, memory problems, attention deficits, word retrieval problems, psychomotor disturbances and a hypersensitivity to sensory stimulation, among others. Once again, the ME/CFS patients' cognitive impairments were substantially, different from those of the healthy controls. Moreover, this cognitive dysfunction may be the result of biochemical and physiological abnormalities in the patients themselves, such as lower cerebral blood flow and reduced grey and white brain matter. As with the other core symptom categories, the cognitive impairments can severely impact the patients' daily life including, their employability and their functional capacity in social environments.

A discussed in Chapter 2, I experienced many of the cognitive manifestations noted in this section. The extreme mental fatigue that I experienced left me in a constant state of mental fog and I consequently, had to slowly make my way through my cognitive world. I also had great difficulty sustaining attention, recalling information, expressing my ideas, processing information and socializing with family and friends. I was uncharacteristically, always forgetful, misplacing things and second guessing my decision making. I further experienced a paucity in my psychomotor skills, and a hypersensitivity to noise, odors, light and extreme temperatures.

Everywhere I turned, I seemed to be facing a new and life limiting cognitive impairment. My inability to simply think and undertake the most basic of motor skills, left this once fairly, competent and somewhat intelligent individual riddled with anxiety and despair, and feeling inept, discouraged and disillusioned.

Orthostatic intolerance (OI)

Orthostatic intolerance (OI) is a clinical condition in which patients' symptoms worsen upon standing or maintaining an upright position. OI can be triggered by the simplest of activities such as standing in line, participating in a low impact exercise, walking, eating, quietly sitting for a prolonged period of time or, exposure to a warm environment, [101]. OI is associated with the patients' overwhelming sense of exhaustion, muscle weakness and need to lie down [102]. OI is typically, ameliorated by recumbency [103]. The severity of the patients' OI symptoms is believed to predict their functional status and ability to live their day-to-day lives [104].

OI is caused by: a) arousal fatigue due to poor sleep quality and quantity, b) oxygenation fatigue due to insufficient oxygen being delivered to the brain and tissues, and c) metabolic fatigue due to the body's cells being unable to transform substrates of energy into useful functions [105].

The symptoms associated with OI are varied and include lightheadedness, dizziness, headaches, nausea, impaired concentration, spatial disorientation, dimming or blurring of vision, dry eyes, sweating, heart palpitations, tremulousness, pain in the left chest and numbness in the feet, legs and arms [22, 106]. Other common OI symptoms include an intolerance to hot or cold weather, shortness of breath, forceful beating of the heart, exercise intolerance, abdominal pain and facial pallor [22, 102]. Finally, OI is associated with a drop-in blood pressure, fainting and "an inability to stand for even a few minutes" [107].

Research has found that the incidence of OI is quite high in ME/CFS patients [108]. In fact, 70% of all patients experience debilitating fatigue, diminished concentration, heart palpitations, dizziness, nausea, tremulousness and visual disturbances [109]. Ninety six percent of patients reported the specific OI symptom of lightheadedness, 96% nausea, 78% abdominal discomfort and 78% blurred vision [110]. Moreover, 61% of patients reported an intolerance to being on their feet, 94% memory or concentration problems, 82% thinking difficulties, 72% exercise intolerance and 65% frequent headaches [89]. Relative to the healthy controls, ME/CFS patients also experienced significantly higher scores of OI, vasomotor (i.e., regulates blood pressure and other homeostatic processes), gastrointestinal, pupillomotor (i.e., changes in the pupil) and sleep problems [111].

Some studies suggest that OI may be the result of a loss of beat-to-beat heart control, blood pressure abnormalities and reduced cerebral blood flow. ME/CFS patients have been found for example, to have a smaller heart cardiothoracic ratio (i.e., heart size) [109], a cardiac contractility deficit of 25.1% [112] and a greater left ventricular work index. In fact, 95% of patients experienced a greater left ventricular work index upon standing, suggesting that their hearts were working harder when they assumed an upright position [108]. Sixty three percent of patients were also found to have blood volume deficits (BVD), as a result of the reduced cerebral blood flow [113]. The BVD, which are in the order of 15.1% [112] and 10.4% [114], can result in the pooling of blood in the legs, abdomen and hands thus, contributing to the patients' OI experiences. The accumulating cardiovascular evidence relating to the loss of beat-to-beat heart control, impaired blood pressure regulation, reduced cerebral blood flow and general autonomic dysfunction (e.g., breathing abnormalities and temperature regulation abnormalities), have led some researchers to posit that ME/CFS patients may be at an increased risk of longer-term cardiovascular problems, such as heart disease [115]. Finally, some researchers suggest that the increased heart rate and the more pronounced systolic blood pressure fall, when patients assume a standing position, may further be related to the cardiovascular deconditioning that is associated with the ME/CFS disease state, as a result of the patients' decreased activity levels [92].

In summary, OI can be triggered by the simplest of activities such as standing, walking or quietly sitting for a prolonged period of time. Once triggered, ME/CFS patients can experience an overwhelming sense of exhaustion, muscle weakness, lightheadedness, dizziness, nausea, spatial disorientation, cognitive difficulties, heart palpitations, shortness of breath and vision problems. Studies suggest that the OI symptoms may be the result of physiological abnormalities, such as a loss of beat-to-beat heart control, impaired blood pressure regulation and decreased cerebral blood flow. Finally, the OI manifestations, which have been both quantified and qualified, can severely limit the patients' ability to fully live their lives.

OI has been a part of my journey too. As outlined in Chapter 2, I experienced many of the cited manifestations such as an inability to stand for any length of time, dizziness, headaches, nausea, spatial disorientation, muscle weakness and tremulousness. I also experienced heart palpitations, labored breathing, sweating, incredible pain in my left chest, and numbness in my face, arms and legs. OI was very, concerning for me particularly in view of these latter symptoms, as I thought that I might be developing a heart problem. In my experience, OI made simple, everyday activities like cooking a simple meal, sitting up to eat a meal, walking, standing and even sitting in the backyard on a warm day extremely, challenging. In many respects, OI was very life limiting!

In concluding this chapter, the research literature has quantitatively and qualitatively confirmed patients' disease experiences. It has also identified five core and four secondary symptom categories that speak to this multi-system disease and the dysfunction that it can cause in patients' lives. The five core symptom categories consist of impaired day-to-day functioning due to the debilitating fatigue, PEM, sleep dysfunction, cognitive impairments and OI while, the secondary symptom categories consist of pain, infection, immune impairments and neuroendocrine manifestations. Each of the five core symptom categories, which are the more universally present and severe in patients' disease experiences, are associated with their own varied and debilitating symptoms and can, in and of themselves, be challenging for patients. Many of the core symptom categories, however, operate in tandem, to varying degrees in the patients' disease experience. The possible accumulation of symptoms, from each of the five core symptom categories plus those of the four secondary symptom categories, only add to the complexity and burden of living with this devastating, complex, multi-system disease.

The research literature cited in this chapter has helped me to understand that ME/CFS, even though it is invisible and sounds rather benign, can be an extremely debilitating and life consuming disease. The numerous, varied, severe and long-lasting symptoms can be life changing! This literature has also provided me with the knowledge that I am not alone in my experiences. In fact, my physical, cognitive and spiritual challenges were all well documented. Moreover, this literature has helped me to appreciate that I am struggling with a devastating, complex, multi-system disease that causes biochemical and physiological dysfunction of the "neurological, immune, endocrine and energy/metabolism systems" [6]. While ME/CFS may be invisible to "others", it is unarguably not "all in the patient's head". ME/CFS and its many manifestations have been scientifically validated. ME/CFS is irrefutably, real!

Now, that we have a deeper understanding of this chronic, invisible, complex, multi-system disease and the extent to which it can challenge and severely impair patients' daily lives, let's have a look at some of the other possible patient outcomes and the prognoses of this disease. Chapter 5 will explore these subject matters.

Chapter 5

OTHER POSSIBLE PATIENT OUTCOMES AND DISEASE PROGNOSES

What lies behind us and what lies before us are tiny matters compared to what lies within us

~ Ralph Waldo Emerson

To enjoy good health, to bring true happiness to one's family, to bring peace to all, one must first discipline and control one's own mind. If a man can control his mind, he can find the way to Enlightenment, and all wisdom and virtue will naturally come to him

~ Buddha

As discussed in Chapter 1, the impacts of ME/CFS can be far reaching, touching the lives of patients, their loved ones, care givers, employers, medical and research communities, and economies at large. The overall burden of ME/CFS is felt at many levels of our society but no more so, than on the daily lives of the patients themselves. In addition to the numerous, varied, relentless and debilitating physical, cognitive and spiritual challenges of this disease, there are a multitude of other possible patient outcomes. Among these outcomes are lifestyle restrictions and social isolation, increased work absences and medical costs, income losses, unemployment, quality of life and longevity concerns, stigmatization and a lack of family, social and medical support [1, 2]. ME/CFS patients are, in fact, "more likely to lose their jobs, possessions and support from friends and family than are people who have other conditions that cause fatigue" [3]. This chapter will seek to shed some light on these other possible patient outcomes. Outcomes that one does not typically, consider when thinking about the effects of a chronic, invisible and debilitating disease. This chapter will also seek to shed some light on the possible prognoses of ME/CFS. As we shall see, the patients' prognoses (i.e., expected timeline for recovery) can also vary, quite substantially, posing further patient challenges and outcomes.

Lifestyle restrictions and social isolation

As previously noted, patients' experiences with ME/CFS vary according to the number, type, severity and duration of their symptoms [4]. The more severe cases, or the higher levels of patient disability, are associated with extreme fatigue, a greater number of physical and cognitive symptoms, poorer physical fitness, poorer sleep quality, and increased mood disorders such as, depression and anxiety [5]. In its more moderate to severe form, ME/CFS can leave once healthy, vital and energetic individuals unable to function and participate in their daily, social, family and work lives [4].

Patients who experience a milder case of ME/CFS often continue to lead relatively normal lives while, individuals who experience a more moderate to severe case can face significant, lifestyle restrictions and social isolation [6]. The individuals who experience a milder case typically, have significantly higher levels of daily uptime and experience less fluctuation in their daily activity levels. In contrast, the more severely impaired individuals face significantly lower levels of daily uptime, are highly functionally impaired in their mobility [7], and face critical reductions both in their activity levels and the complexity of the activities that they are able to undertake [8, 9]. These individuals also experience high fluctuations in their daily activities, are only able to participate in low intensity activities such as sitting quietly or watching television [10], and face severe activity restrictions at home, work and in their social environments [11, 12]. Moreover, an estimated one quarter of all patients are so severely impaired that they are bedridden, virtually unable to do anything, and dependent on others for their daily care [11, 12]. These individuals are also characterized by extremely high levels of daily fatigue, high levels of passive activities and severe mobility and daily activity impairments [13]. In its more severe form, ME/CFS can consume the patient's life [3].

The Canadian data on patient activity restrictions (Figure 6), demonstrate the substantial lifestyle restrictions that ME/CFS can impose on patients' lives. Approximately, 74% of ME/CFS patients for example, experienced activity restrictions at home, 67% in other activities (including social activities) and 59% at work while, 36% faced productivity losses. When compared to other chronic and disabling disorders such as multiple chemical sensitivities (MCS) and fibromyalgia (FMS), the ME/CFS patients reported higher levels of activity restrictions. The only exceptions to this were for FMS, which slightly exceeded the ME/CFS patients' activity restrictions at work (61% verses 59%) and at home (79% verses 74%). The contrast between the ME/CFS and no MUPS patients' activity restrictions, however, is quite stark. Only 19% of the no MUPS patients (e.g., cancer, diabetes or heart disease), reported activity restrictions at home (verses 74%), 18% in other activities (vs. 67%), 14% at work (vs. 59%) and 5% faced productivity losses (vs. 36%). On the basis of this data ME/CFS, with few exceptions, imposes higher levels of activity restrictions on patients' home, work and social lives as well as, on their productivity.

Increased work absences, unemployment, reduced income and higher medical costs

Increased work absences, unemployment, reduced income and higher medical costs are other possible ME/CFS patient outcomes. In terms of the work absences, estimates suggest that more than half of all ME/CFS patients were not able to work at all and that nearly two thirds were limited in their ability to work [8, 12]. Of these patients, more than half were on disability or temporary sick leave, less than 35% were able to work full-time and 40% worked on a part time basis [11]. In a more recent study, 82% of patients were unable to work or attend school on a full-time basis, 15% were unable to work more than 30 hours a week and 47% were permanently disabled [15]. The unemployment rates among patients are estimated to range from 35-69% [15].

Figure 6: Prevalence of activity restriction/productivity loss due to chronic illness, by medically unexplained physical symptoms (MUPS) status, household population aged 25 to 75, Canada 2014

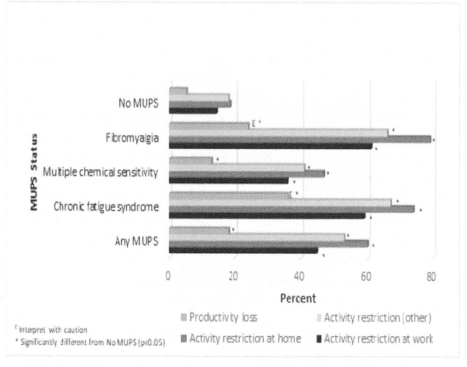

Source: Canadian Community Health Survey, 2014; cited in Park and Gilmour (2017) [48]. No MUPS includes disorders such as diabetes, cancer, heart disease and asthma.

In examining the Canadian ME/CFS labor force data (Figure 7), one notes that approximately 35% of Canadian patients continued to have a job, 42% did not have a job and 23% were permanently unable to work. These figures are again, in sharp contrast to the no MUPS patients (e.g., cancer, heart disease or diabetes) as 71% of the no MUPS continued to have a job (verses 35%), 26% did not have a job (verses 42%) and only 3%

(verses 23%) were permanently unable to work. Relative to the FMS and MCS patients, the ME/CFS patients, once again, reported higher rates of not having a job (40% and 39% vs. 42%, respectively) and of being permanently unable to work (20% and 8% versus 23%, respectively). The ME/CFS patients also reported the lowest rates of having a job (38% and 53% versus 35%, respectively). On the basis of this data, ME/CFS imposes higher labour force activity restrictions than the other chronic and fatiguing diseases.

Figure 7: Labour force status, by medically unexplained physical symptoms (MUPS) status, household population aged 25 to 75, Canada, 2014

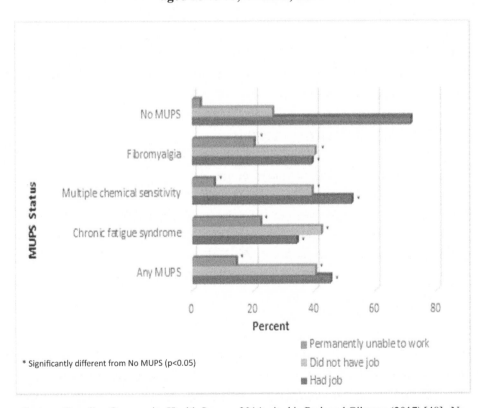

Source: Canadian Community Health Survey, 2014; cited in Park and Gilmour (2017) [48]. No MUPS includes disorders such as diabetes, cancer, heart disease and asthma.

In terms of reduced incomes, in the U.S., the annual household income loss is an estimated $20,000 per ME/CFS patient [14] while, the household productivity loss is an estimated 37% [16]. Facing the loss of one's income is very, challenging but to complicate matters further, many patients also face increased medical costs. The annual direct medical costs per patient in the U.S. range from an estimated $2,342 for previously undiagnosed patients to $8,675 for diagnosed patients [17]. Another estimate suggests that the direct medical costs are more in the range of $3,286 per patient [18]. The annual direct (e.g., office visits, medical tests and medications) and indirect (e.g., loss of income and productivity) costs per patient, however, are an estimated $30,860. [19]. The increased work absences, reduced earning capacity, loss of employment and increased medical costs can have further impacts on the patients' lives. These impacts include the loss of the patients' financial independence, home, personal possessions and overall sense of health and well-being. The labor force and financial impacts of ME/CFS, like the disease itself, can be extremely challenging, burdensome and life changing for patients.

Quality of life and longevity concerns

ME/CFS can also impose quality of life and longevity concerns for patients. In addition to the physical, cognitive and spiritual challenges of this disease, many patients experience some form of psychological dysfunction such as depression, anxiety, stress and irritability [4]. In fact, an estimated 45% of all patients experience some form of psychological dysfunction [20]. These psychological disorders, which are believed to be related to the stress of living with the numerous, unexplained and debilitating symptoms, can drastically impact the patients' quality of life and only add to the challenges of living with ME/CFS [21]. Moreover, depression is of major concern for patients as it impacts not only their quality of life but potentially, their longevity too [22]. When compared to individuals with other chronic conditions, ME/CFS patients experience much higher rates of depression and sadly, the depression can lead to suicide [4, 12]. In fact, when compared to the general population, ME/CFS patients tend to experience much higher rates of suicide [4]. So, while ME/CFS itself is typically, not considered a fatal disease, suicide can be a real concern for some patients.

Cancer and heart disease can also impose quality of life and longevity concerns for patients. In fact, cancer, heart disease and suicide are the most common causes of death among patients [3]. The chronic activation of the immune system, associated with ME/CFS, is believed to play a role in the patients' increased risk of cancer [23] while, the loss of beat-to-beat heart control, impaired blood pressure regulation and autonomic dysfunction that have been found in some patients, as discussed in Chapter 4, may put these patients at an increased risk of heart disease [24]. Raised levels of oxidative stress, low grade inflammation and increased arterial stiffness may also be responsible for this increased cardiovascular risk [25]. Finally, a progressive degeneration of end organs, most particularly that of the heart and pancreas, have also resulted in some patients' early death [26]. When compared to the general populace, ME/CFS patients also tend to experience much higher, early death rates [27]. In final analysis, while ME/CFS is not considered a fatal disease, it can pose the risk of premature death [3, 28].

Stigmatization and a lack of family, social and medical support

Other possible ME/CFS patient outcomes include stigmatization and a lack of family, social and medical support. In terms of patient stigmatization, some researchers argue that the term "ME/CFS" itself may be at the root of and contribute to this stigmatization. These researchers posit that "ME/CFS" may conjure images of a benign disease and thus, trivialize both the disease itself and its impact on the patients' lives [3]. This stigmatization may thus contribute to "others" (e.g., family members, friends, caregivers and medical personnel) questioning if patients are malingering, wondering if ME/CFS is real and judging patients for having the disease [3].

In a similar vein, the lack of family, social and medical support that many patients experience frequently, stems from "others'" beliefs that ME/

CFS is caused by factors that are internal to the patient. In other words, the disease was brought on by the patients themselves [28]. This belief can result in "others" blaming the patients for having ME/CFS, harboring negative feelings towards them [28] and being highly, critical of them [29]. "Others'" beliefs can also result in the patients' health condition being judged as fake, their health concerns being dismissed and them facing harsh judgements, public disapproval and shame for having this disease [7]. The beliefs and judgements of others can further lead to patients feeling alone, misunderstood and unsupported [7]. Moreover, they can lead to poorer, patient medical outcomes. Outcomes that include increased levels of fatigue and depression and reduced emotional and psychosocial well-being [30]. In many respects, the beliefs, judgements and behaviors of "others", can greatly add to the patients' challenges and burden of living with ME/CFS.

Having to constantly cope with the numerous and relentless physical, cognitive and spiritual challenges of ME/CFS as well as, the judgements and behaviors of others, can create a great deal of psychological upheaval for the patients. This upheaval can lead to high levels of patient anxiety, stress and uncertainty [31]. It can also lead to patients struggling with their sense of self. Many patients for example, struggle with who they once were, who they are now and how they need to rebuild their life [32, 33, 34]. In addition, many patients have great difficulty accepting their "new" self and their "new" life [31]. A crisis of identity is not uncommon [31]. The psychological upheaval imposed by this disease can be relentless.

Understandably, it can be difficult for significant "others" (e.g., family members and care givers) to live and cope with their loved one's diagnosis. Knowing that ME/CFS can be a long-term illness, and witnessing the debilitating and life changing effects that ME/CFS is having on their loved one, can add to the distress of the significant "others", impacting their life and sense of well-being too [29]. The burden of living with ME/CFS is felt by patients, their loved ones and care givers alike [35]. ME/CFS can be challenging and life changing for all concerned.

The lack of medical support that many patients experience further includes a dismissiveness of their health concerns, negative interactions with and exposure to hostile attitudes from the medical community [32] as well as, being subjected to treatment strategies that exacerbate their symptoms [36, 37]. This lack of support, when compared to the support that individuals experiencing other chronic illnesses receive, is more prevalent among ME/CFS patients [35] and may be due, in part, to the medical community's lack of awareness and knowledge about this disease [32]. Less than 1/3 of all medical schools for example, include ME/CFS in their curriculum and only 40% of the medical textbooks include some information about ME/CFS [38, 39]. There have been repeated calls for improvements to be made to educational resources as a means of facilitating patients, their loved ones, health care providers and society at large, in better understanding this disease and its debilitating effects on patients' lives [40].

The sociocultural environment is very, important to a society's understanding of a disease and so too, is the research funding allocated to it. Research can lead to a better understanding of ME/CFS, to advancing its diagnostics and to developing more effective treatment options [3, 40]. The research funding allocated to ME/CFS however, appears to be somewhat lacking. Relative to the funding allocated to other chronic diseases such as HIV/AIDS, lupus and multiple sclerosis, the U.S. National Institute of Health's (NIH) funding for ME/CFS is nominal particularly, in view of ME/CFS' prevalence (Table 6). The prevalence of ME/CFS far exceeds that of lupus and multiple sclerosis by 2-3 times and yet, the research funding is substantially less, $5 million verses $99 and $102 million, respectively. Moreover, while ME/CFS and HIV/AIDS are comparable in disease prevalence, the spending per ME/CFS patient is only $5.00 compared to $2,482. for HIV/AIDS. An estimated 25-fold increase in annual ME/CFS research funding is believed necessary, to be commensurate with its disease burden (i.e., number of people affected by an illness and the associated disability and early death rates) [41].

Table 6: 2014 U.S. National Institute of Health (NIH)
Funding and Prevalence of Selected Diseases

Disease area	Funding (Millions)	U.S. Prevalence	$ Spending per patient
HIV/AIDs	$2,978	1,200,000	$2,482
Lupus	$99	350,000	$283
Multiple sclerosis	$102	400,000	$255
ME/CFS	$5	1,060,000	$5

Source: Dimmock, Mirin and Jason, 2016 [39].

Fair ME/CFS research funding, commensurate with its disease burden, is an estimated $190 million a year [40]. There thus remains a "massive shortfall" in ME/CFS research funding [42]. From my perspective, an increased level of ME/CFS research funding may go a long way to creating a better understanding of this disease, to reducing its stigma and to increasing social and medical support for patients.

I can certainly relate to some of the patients' reported feelings of stigmatization and judgement from "others". Over the years, I have heard comments like "Deb, you are not easy on yourself" possible implication, you did something to bring this disease on or, "you can't be that tired" possible implication, it really cannot be that bad or, "get up and get going" possible implication, just push through it, you are limiting yourself or, "you look so healthy" possible implication, you are exaggerating your condition. In my experience, people often have little understanding of this disease and cannot fathom: a) the profound levels of fatigue, b) the significant need for sleep and rest, c) the body's lack of stamina and inability to recover after nominal exertion, d) the many and varied symptoms and e) the devastating impacts that ME/CFS can have on a patient's daily life – mind, body and soul.

Over the years, I have become more reluctant to share my ME/CFS diagnosis with "others". I too, on occasion, felt "others" blame and my shame for having this disease. I have also felt judged (e.g., I don't visibly see any symptoms so what is really going on with you), dismissed (e.g., Deb, we all struggle with fatigue) and stigmatized (e.g., it is only fatigue). I understand, ME/CFS is an invisible and misunderstood disease and oft times, as individuals, when something is not visibly obvious or is not within our realm of personal experiences, we can have difficulty perceiving and understanding it. However, the judgement, stigmatization and dismissiveness can have unintended, negative consequences for the patients' health and overall sense of well-being. In my experience, the psychological upheaval, in conjunction with the numerous, varied and relentless challenges imposed by this disease, could be unbearable.

The Prognoses

The prognoses of ME/CFS, or the expected timeline for recovery, can also vary, quite substantially among patients. Generally speaking, individuals who experience an acute onset of the disease, such as through an infection or a virus, typically, improve within two years. Individuals who experience a more, gradual onset however, are more likely to experience a longer duration of the illness [43, 44]. ME/CFS can be a short, a prolonged and continuous illness or, one that returns in episodes for periods of 6 months or longer, with relapses occurring years after the onset of the disease [43, 44]. On average, the ME/CFS recovery rate is between 3-7 years, with some patients feeling better within 6 months and others, continuing to be ill 20 years later [11]. The median length of ME/CFS is 12.5 years [15].

While some patients may experience symptom improvement, a full recovery (i.e., restoration to the premorbid level of health) is seldom achieved in adults [44] including, for those individuals who participate in treatment programs such as cognitive behavioral therapy (CBT) and graded exercise therapy (GET) (to be discussed in Chapter 6) [45]. It is estimated that 0-6% [26] and 0-12% [44] of all adults may experience a full recovery. Predictors for a full recovery include the patients' age, gender, severity and duration of symptoms, beliefs about the illness, cognitive and behavioral responses, levels of anxiety and depression, and work and social adjustment [25]. An accurate prognosis cannot, therefore, be predicted with any certainty [26, 44].

As a full recovery is seldom achieved in adults, many patients will continue to be symptomatic, have reduced levels of function and may face relapses years after remission [44, 46]. In one study that followed patients over a 5-year period, 27.5% of all patients reported an improvement in their symptoms at the first-year follow-up while, 50-65% reported little to no change in their condition, even after participating in a treatment program. At the 5-year follow-up however, 84.4% of all patients reported that they continued to suffer from ME/CFS while, 17% reported a substantial deterioration in their health over that 5-year period [47]. In another 5-year study, patients' work disability rates increased from 77% to 91% [48]. Finally, in a more recent study, 96% of patients experienced little improvement in their symptoms over a 10-year time-period [15]. Prognoses for adults are generally, regarded as "poor and current care [as] limited" [49].

In summation, the numerous, varied, relentless and debilitating symptoms that accompany ME/CFS can drastically alter patients' lives. When one adds the other possible patient outcomes to the disease state, the impact of ME/CFS can be even, more burdensome. Patients run the risk of not only being deeply challenged by ME/CFS but, they can also face severe lifestyle restrictions, social isolation, a loss of income, employment and financial independence, quality of life and longevity concerns, a loss of self-identity, a lack of family, social and medical support, and challenging relationships. Moreover, prognoses tend to be poor in adults. In light of these poorer prognoses, these other possible outcomes may be long term and quite possibly, even last a lifetime. ME/CFS can inarguably, be a grueling, relentless and life changing disease that can devastate patients' lives on so many levels.

Much needs to be done to enhance "others'" awareness and understanding of this disease, including increased levels of research funding. Ongoing research is extremely important to understanding, diagnosing, treating and finding a cure for this disease. While the prognoses for ME/CFS is currently regarded as poor for adults, with enhanced funding and ongoing research, patients and their loved ones can expect that more effective treatments and a cure for this disease will be found.

As I mentioned at the outset of this chapter, many of these other possible patient outcomes are not typically, what one considers when thinking about the effects of a chronic, invisible and debilitating disease. This is extremely unfortunate, as these other possible outcomes are extensive and very impactful. The research literature presented in this chapter has certainly helped me to better understand these "broader" patient outcomes and my experiences with them. I too, faced severe lifestyle restrictions, social isolation, the loss of my career, a crisis of identity, difficulties in accepting my "new" self and my "new" life, psychological dysfunction, concerns over my health outcome, and stigmatization and judgement from others. In many respects, this literature has been like a healing balm – soothing my experiences with the "broader" impacts of this disease and adding to my self-understanding. In final analysis, this literature has helped me to more deeply appreciate that patients face not only the varied, relentless and devastating physical, cognitive and spiritual challenges associated with this disease but, they can also face the varied, relentless and devastating socio-cultural and economic challenges as well. The burden of living with ME/CFS is multi-faceted!

Now that we have examined some of the other possible patient outcomes and the prognoses of this disease, let's take a look at some of the treatments for ME/CFS. Chapter 6 will explore the various ME/CFS treatments.

Chapter 6

TREATING ME/CFS

When you reach the end of your rope, tie a knot in it and hang on
~ Franklin D. Roosevelt

Out of suffering have emerged the strongest souls; the most massive
characters are seared with scars

~ Kahlil Gibran

In the initial phases of this disease, I had difficulty understanding how some individuals were able to recover their health within a short period of time while, I remained bedridden and unable to sustain any amount of activity, for the longest time. I desperately wanted to recover my health, to return to my career and to, once again, fully live my life. I, therefore, turned to the ME/CFS treatment literature, in the hopes of understanding what treatments might facilitate my recovery. In doing so, I soon came to realize that, according to the research literature, there is no known treatment that results in a cure for this disease [1, 2]. Treatments, therefore, seek to improve the patients' symptoms, their management of the disease and their quality of life [1, 2]. Among the treatments that may be of benefit to patients are the "rehabilitative type" such as cognitive behavioral therapy (CBT) and graded exercise therapy (GET), medications, a healthy diet, vitamins and supplements, and "other" treatments such as massage therapy, yoga and physiotherapy [3, 4]. Until recently, CBT and GET have been regarded as the more effective of these treatments. They were, in fact, recommended by the U.K.'s NICE and the U.S.'s CDC, for patients experiencing a mild to moderate case of ME/CFS [4, 5]. However, their effectiveness and safety are currently being questioned [4, 6]. This chapter will sequentially, examine each of the above noted treatments and provide a more fulsome discussion of the CBT and GET debate.

Cognitive behavioral therapy (CBT)

CBT is a non-drug, psychological based approach that seeks to improve the patients' symptoms and quality of life through cognitive and behavioral changes. Some of the cognitive processes that may play a role in perpetuating the patients' symptoms are: a) their perceptions that the fatigue is difficult to influence and b) their focus on the fatigue's debilitating effects on their life [7]. Through CBT, patients can change these cognitive processes by developing a better understanding of their symptoms, accepting the disease and the limitations that it imposes on their life [9, 10], and developing strategies that can ultimately, improve their quality of life [2, 4, 8].

CBT seeks to support ME/CFS patients by helping them learn how to: a) listen to their body and not push themselves into situations of overexertion and relapse (i.e., the "push-crash" cycle), b) reduce their concerns about the mistakes that they make, c) cope better with their depression and mood disorders (e.g., anxiety, guilt and anger) and d) develop a more positive outlook on their life [11, 12, 13]. Moreover, patients have opportunities to address their fears, their embarrassment about having ME/CFS and "others'" judgements and reactions towards them [14, 15]. Strategies such as positive reframing, learning how to better plan their activities and reducing their reliance on behavioral disengagement (e.g., removing themselves from social activities) are all key to enhancing the patients' quality of life as well as, their work and social adjustment [2, 11, 16].

CBT can also help ME/CFS patients develop better stress management skills (SMS). As discussed in Chapter 3, some patients experience lower levels of cortisol and consequently, experience more fatigue and PEM. The cortisol awakening response (CAR) has been identified as a "marker of endocrine dysregulation", relevant to the patients' fatigue and PEM experiences. Through SMS, patients can learn how to manage their CAR, improve their cortisol levels and experience less fatigue [17]. Other studies, however, have suggested that the patients' lower levels of cortisol may not only be responsible for the persistence of their fatigue and PEM but, may also be responsible for the patients' poorer responses to CBT, as will be discussed shortly [18, 19].

CBT has certainly been a welcome part of my treatment approach. I have found my CBT sessions to be very, helpful as I am able to freely share my experiences with this disease and its devastating effects on my life. I am also able to unabashedly express my disillusionment, grief, anxiety and despair. My psychologist offers me a safe place, with no judgement. She also offers me validation, empathy and sound counsel. In my CBT sessions, I was asked to address the fact, as will be discussed in Chapter 7, that maybe my health status is as good as it is going to get, that maybe I need to be more accepting of my life as it is and that maybe, this is my "new normal". In sharing my experiences and sentiments as well as, addressing some of the "harsher" realities of ME/CFS, I believe that I am now more accepting of this disease's challenges and limitations on my life. I am also more cognizant of my need to better plan my activities so that I do not fall into the "push-crash" cycle, to not get upset with myself when I make mistakes, to take "others" judgements and reactions in stride and to try to see my life in a more positive light. I firmly, believe that CBT has been conducive to my overall sense of health and well-being. My trust in and "partnership" with my psychologist have added greatly to my positive CBT experiences. I am extremely thankful that she has been there for me during this very, difficult time in my life.

Graded exercise therapy (GET)

GET is another non-drug therapy that is used in the treatment of ME/CFS. In GET, patients are encouraged to gradually return to their physical activities through supportive behavioral changes. Through tailored, light to moderate exercise activities, patients are helped to move from their more basic activity levels, to increased physical functioning [4, 7]. GET typically, works best when combined with CBT [4, 7].

GET seeks to strike the right balance between the patients' over and under activity, by ceasing exercise activities before fatigue and illness set in. Patients are encouraged by their physical/rehabilitative therapist to initially, start with minimal activity such as 3-5 minutes of exercise a day [4]. Patients are also asked to be mindful of their need for rest, a key element in patient management, and to adjust their schedules and activity levels according to their daily energy peaks and valleys. Patient feedback and the mutual planning of activities are critical to the success of GET [4, 20].

GET may not however, be beneficial for all patients, most particularly, those patients who are severely affected by ME/CFS. For such patients, any form of exercise – no matter how nominal – can bring on profound levels of fatigue and intensify many of their other symptoms. In fact, some of the more severely affected patients may only be able to sustain exercise activities for one minute at a time and even then, they may suffer an exacerbation of their many symptoms [4, 6, 7]. Moreover, some patients, when participating in GET, experience reduced maximum heart rates while, other patients experience significantly, impaired oxygen consumption levels (as discussed in Chapter 4). The research, therefore, cautions that patients not, be pushed beyond their physical capabilities as "exercises that would be aerobic for healthy individuals, may be anaerobic for [ME/CFS] patients" [21].

GET was initially, a part of my treatment plan as well. Shortly after my diagnosis, as a means of trying to recover my energy levels, I participated in a rehabilitative, physical exercise program. I personally, found the program to be rather aggressive as I was expected to complete a schedule of activities, regardless of how I was feeling. I often felt pushed beyond my physical capabilities and had great difficulty completing the exercises as I was fatigued, nauseated, weak and disoriented. These experiences were a big change for me, given my former athleticism. Upon returning home, I faced an exacerbation of my symptoms and required a lot of sleep, for days later. In my experience, GET intensified my symptoms and left me feeling very, discouraged. My doctors subsequently, recommended that I cease my participation in this rehabilitative program. It is quite possible that the rehabilitative therapist did not fully understand ME/CFS and the impact that exercise, including nominal exercise, can have on a patient. He may, therefore, have pushed me beyond my physical capabilities and beyond any of the rehabilitative benefits of such a program. Regardless, a physical rehabilitation program was not helpful in restoring my energy and physical activity levels. To this day, nominal exercise intensifies my level of fatigue and my many other symptoms. Exercise thus, continues to be anaerobic rather than rejuvenating and invigorating for me.

The CBT and GET debate

CBT and GET have long-been viewed as the more effective of the ME/CFS treatment protocols and both approaches have been deemed valuable in improving patients' symptoms and quality of life. Thirty one percent of patients for example, reported symptom improvement post CBT and GET [24], and 18% reported a full recovery following CBT [23]. However, more recent studies have noted that while a minority of patients may fully recover, most patients do not profit at all from either of these treatments [24, 25]. Hence the debate.

Some researchers are now questioning the effectiveness of CBT and GET. They posit that CBT yields little to moderate effectiveness and that both CBT and GET fail to provide clinically, significant outcomes [26, 27]. Yet other researchers argue that CBT and GET may be detrimental to the patients' health and safety [25, 28, 29, 30]. One such study noted that many patients experienced significant deterioration following CBT and GET [31] while, another study found that GET was associated with high rates of patient harm [25]. Seventy percent of patients for example, reported that GET made their symptoms worse while, 73% reported that CBT did not provide symptom relief [29]. Moreover, while some adult patients may experience some recovery and no longer maintain a ME/CFS diagnosis, most patients are unlikely to return to their premorbid levels of health, even after CBT and GET [32]. Finally, the effects of CBT and GET in improving the patients' quality of life are believed to be small [1, 12] and to date, no treatment intervention has proven itself effective in restoring the patients' ability to work [23].

On the basis of the foregoing findings, some researchers have stated that there is limited evidence to suggest that CBT and GET lead to symptom improvement and recovery, and that statements to the contrary may be misleading to patients and clinicians alike [12]. These findings have also led the ME Association to recommend that both the NICE and CDC remove CBT and GET from their treatment protocols [29]. In 2017, the CDC removed these protocols from its website [33, 34, 35]. Other global providers of clinical ME/CFS guidance have also been invited to revisit their practices of including CBT and GET in their treatment protocols [36]. So, while CBT and GET may be of benefit to some patients, they may be detrimental to others. As will be discussed shortly, there is growing support for ME/CFS treatments to be individualized.

Medications

There is presently, no effective ME/CFS drug therapy [37] and no one particular, medication that is specifically approved for the treatment of this disease. In fact, medications play only a minor role in the management of ME/CFS and are regarded as indirect treatments [4, 6, 38].

Of the medications that may be of benefit to patients are those that treat the pain, sleep disorders, depression and panic disorders [6]. Tylenol, aspirin and non-steroidal anti-inflammatory drugs (NSAIDS) such as Advil, Motrin and Aleve may help patients with their symptoms of pain, swelling and fever [6, 38]. Antidepressants, on the other hand, may improve patients' sleep related disorders and relieve their depression while, anti-anxiety drugs may help patients with their panic disorders. It should be noted however, that while antidepressants may help some patients, they have had varying degrees of success in other patients. Some ME/CFS patients for example, cannot tolerate the higher doses of anti-depressants commonly used to treat depression [4] while, other patients experience unwanted side effects such as, a worsening of their other symptoms [39]. Antidepressants may, therefore, not be effective in treating all patients' symptoms of depression [3, 4, 38]. Prescribed sleep medications have also been found to be helpful to some patients while, worsening other patients' sleep related disorders [40, 41]. Similarly, medications that seek to stimulate patients' central nervous system or energy levels, such as hormones and adrenaline, while helpful to some patients, may cause a hypersensitivity and a "push-crash" cycle in other patients (i.e., over-exertion and relapse). This "push-crash" cycle can result in patients experiencing increased fatigue levels and a worsening of their other symptoms [6].

Gamma globulin, which contains human antibodies to organisms that cause infection, may help boost some patients' immune functions while Ampligen, a drug that stimulates the immune system and possesses antiviral properties, may improve some patients' mental functions. Fludrocortisone may help some patients with their neurally-mediated hypotension (NMH) (https://medical-dictionary.thefree dictionary.com/ chronic+fatigue+syndrome) while, Rituximab may reduce some patients fatigue levels [42]. Finally, increased sodium intake may be beneficial in treating some patients' OI symptoms [43].

Of the ME/CFS medications, the more commonly used are for patients' sleep related disorders (62%), pain, inflammation and muscle spasms (52%), thyroid function/other endocrine/hormonal issues (46%), anxiety, depression or general mental health (36%) and digestive or gastrointestinal concerns such as, irritable bowel (35%) [44]. As noted above, many patients experience unwanted side effects and a hypersensitivity to customary doses of medications [44]. As a result of the patients' unique responses to medications and treatments, the range and severity of their disease symptoms, and their own, unique biological needs, researchers are calling for ME/CFS treatments to be individualized [4, 25].

I can certainly relate to the hypersensitivity and unwanted side effects from certain medications. Prior to my ME/CFS diagnosis, I had been taking numerous medications to help with my chronic vertigo including, medications that sought to stimulate my energy levels and address my sleep related disorders and depression. However, about six to eight months into my journey with ME/CFS, I would frequently hear my inner voice say "I don't want to take these medications any more". I continued to take them, believing that they were of benefit to me until one day, I heard my inner voice shout "Stop it! I don't want these medications – they are making me sick". I spoke with my primary doctor, my GP, about this experience and on her recommendation, I immediately ceased taking the medications. My body had seemingly, developed an intolerance, a hypersensitivity or negative side effects to medications that I had been taking for years.

Throughout the first couple of years following my ME/CFS diagnosis, I continued to try other medications to improve my sleep related disorders, address my anxiety and mood disorders, and increase my energy levels but, my body rebuked them too. I took hormones for example, to address my night sweats, anti-anxiety medications to help with my anxiety, and anti-depressants to help with my depression but, to no avail. I also tried liver and kidney detoxes to help increase my overall energy levels but, I soon discovered that I was highly, sensitive to them too. Finally, I tried adrenaline to increase my energy levels but, I experienced the "push-crash" cycle and relapsed quite badly into fatigue and malaise. In my experience, even a cup of coffee or a caffeine boost from a soft drink, sufficiently stimulated my energy levels and would subsequently, leave me in the "push-crash" cycle. I was extremely hypersensitive! On the basis of my experiences with CBT, GET and medications, I certainly understand the research community's call for treatments to be individualized. Fortunately, my GP invited me to heed my body's wisdom, did not give up on me and to this day, provides me with excellent medical care.

A healthy diet, vitamins and supplements

A balanced and nutritional diet, eaten at regular times and supplemented with water, vitamins and minerals have also been found to be of benefit to ME/CFS patients' overall health [23]. A diet that includes fruits, vegetables, whole grains, low fat or fat-free milk products, lean meats, poultry, fish, beans, eggs and nuts, may further facilitate patients in better meeting their general health requirements [4, 45].

Among the vitamins and supplements that may be of benefit to patients are magnesium (for fatigue and muscle spasms), evening primrose and fish oil (for general health), Vitamin C, E and B complex (natural antioxidants and antihistamines that can help with allergies and the immune system) and grape seed extract (for pain) [15, 46]. Vitamins A, C, B12 and E may also improve patients' immune and mental functions while herbs such as astragalus, echinacea, essiac, garlic, ginseng, gingko, shiitake mushroom extract, borage seed oil and quercetin may improve patients' immune functions [4]. Melatonin and calcium have also shown some success in helping patients with their sleep related problems [4] while, Quinine may help patients with their muscle cramps, baclofen lioresal with their muscle spasms and CO-enzyme 10 with their muscle energy performance [37]. Moreover, probiotics may help some patients with their irritable bowel syndrome (IBS), ginger with their nausea, and cinnarizine/sturgeon with their dizziness [34]. Finally, zinc and magnesium may help patients with their memory and energy levels, and Comfrey with their inflammation [4].

Part of my ME/CFS treatment journey has also included visits with an "environmental" medical doctor for an assessment of my possible food allergies and environmental sensitivities. As we know, food allergies and environmental sensitivities can also trigger symptoms of extreme fatigue, nausea, weakness and general malaise. My GP, therefore, believed that a consultation with an environmental doctor might be an important strategy in alleviating some of my symptoms and improving my overall health. Through these visits, I discovered that I did indeed have a number of food allergies and environmental sensitivities. In understanding what they are, I am now more mindful of them and have developed strategies to address them. In the case of my food allergies, I have either totally, eliminated certain foods from my diet or only consume them on occasion, as recommended. In so doing, I have found some overall relief. In terms of my environmental sensitivities, I am careful and attempt to avoid them wherever possible. It was in these visits that I also discovered my extreme sensitivities to adrenaline and liver and kidney detoxs – in effect, treatments that sought to stimulate my energy levels. I, like other ME/CFS patients, was highly, sensitive to and experienced the "push-crash" cycle as a result of these energy stimulating treatments. Finally, I discovered that I am highly, sensitive to magnesium glycinate, a supplement for body pain.

Revisiting my diet and nutritional needs has been an important part of my treatment journey. Being conscious of eating a balanced and nutritional diet, removing certain foods and limiting my caffeine intake for example, have all been helpful to me. On my GP's recommendation, I have also added vitamins and supplements such as vitamin C, D, B12, Omega oils, calcium, ubiquinol, Q-10, magnesium and probiotics to my regime. Moreover, I have found that increased salt intake helps with my low blood pressure and light headedness, and melatonin with my sleep related problems, when I am not overly tired. If I am overly tired however, melatonin is not effective. Finally, when I am feeling more run down than usual, I take essiac, echinacea or astragalus to boost my immune system and hopefully, ward off a cold or flu. I have found that colds and flus really exacerbate my ME/CFS symptoms. All of these strategies, while not eradicating my ME/CFS symptoms, have provided some welcome relief and have contributed to my overall sense of health and well-being.

Other ME/CFS treatments

A number of "other" treatments have been identified as beneficial to ME/CFS patients. These treatments are not however, recommended as primary ME/CFS treatment strategies [4]. Among these treatments are those that relieve some of the stress and pain associated with ME/CFS such as, biofeedback, deep breathing, massage therapy, meditation, yoga and muscle relaxation techniques [4, 23]. Magnetic pulsers, warm baths, physiotherapy and acupuncture have also shown some benefit in addressing patients' pain concerns while, aromatherapy has shown some benefit in helping patients with their sleep related disorders [4, 23]. Finally, soothing music may reduce patients' anxiety levels, and walking and bright light therapy may help reduce their reactive depression, which frequently results from the patients' reduced functions and social isolation [23].

Traditional Chinese medicine (TCM) such as Chinese herbal medicines, yoga, acupuncture, qigong, moxibustion and acupoint application, have also shown some effectiveness in alleviating patients' fatigue symptoms [47]. Finally, in addition to relieving some of the patients' stress and pain, yoga has shown some effectiveness in improving patients' balance problems [23].

Over the years, I have found a number of these "other" treatments to be of benefit to me as well. Among these are massage therapy, acupuncture, physiotherapy, magnetic pulsers and warm baths. All of these treatments have helped to relieve some of the pain and muscle spasms in my legs, back and neck. Furthermore, warm baths, soothing music and aromatherapy have helped to facilitate my sleep. When I am overly tired however, none of these latter strategies are effective. Finally, walking and bright light therapy have helped with my reactive depression.

Before leaving this chapter, I would like to mention that vaccines and surgeries have been found to exacerbate some patients' symptoms and trigger relapses [25]. I have certainly, found this to be the case with me as well. In terms of vaccines, I had been taking an annual flu shot for many years, as a means of warding off colds and flus, reducing their severity and duration and potentially, reducing the severity and number of my chronic vertigo episodes. Subsequent to my ME/CFS diagnosis however, I noticed that these vaccines left me extremely fatigued, malaised and bedridden for 6-10 days after. I do continue to have an annual flu vaccine though, as I believe that the benefits far outweigh a potentially, severe flu season and the subsequent, triggering of severe episodes of ME/CFS. In terms of surgeries, the septoplasty that I underwent to facilitate my breathing and ultimately, improve my sleep related disorders (as discussed in Chapter 4), also left me very fatigued and malaised for months after. I could not seem to get back up on my feet after the surgery. It is as though any added stress to my body, whether through vaccines, surgery or colds and flus, only act to intensify my ME/CFS condition. Finally, identifying which treatment approaches were most beneficial to me involved some trial and error. Again, I would like to reiterate that I am not advocating a specific approach, I am simply stating what my ME/CFS experiences have been.

In concluding this chapter, there is presently no known treatment that results in a cure for ME/CFS. The treatment goals are, therefore, to improve the patients' symptoms, their self-management of the disease and ultimately, their quality of life. Among the treatment strategies that have been identified as being of benefit to patients are CBT and GET, medications, a healthy diet, vitamins and supplements, and "other" treatments such as massage therapy, physiotherapy and yoga. As noted, there is growing support for treatment approaches to be individualized, as treatments that may be beneficial to some patients, may be detrimental to others. Patients may, therefore, need to work closely with their doctor/s to determine which of the treatment approaches are most beneficial to them. In final analysis, many of the above noted treatments, while not providing a cure for ME/

CFS, may improve the patients' symptoms and overall sense of health and well-being. I remain hopeful however, that more effective treatments and a cure will be found for this debilitating and life changing disease in the not too distant future.

Now that I have presented an account of my journey with ME/CFS from the physical, cognitive and spiritual points of view as well as, my journey through the research literature, in search of a deeper understanding of this disease and my experiences with it, I would now like to briefly share some of my reflections along the way. Reflections that have helped me to make sense of my journey with ME/CFS and move forward with my "new" life. Chapter 7 will enumerate these reflections.

Chapter 7

REFLECTIONS ALONG THE WAY

*Nothing splendid has ever been achieved except by those who dared
believe that something inside of them was superior to circumstance*
~ *Bruce Barton*

*Bad things do happen; how I respond to them defines my character
and the quality of my life. I can choose to sit in perpetual sadness,
immobilized by the gravity of my loss, or I can choose to rise from
the pain and treasure the most precious gift I have – life itself*
~ *Walter Anderson*

I was one of those individuals who thought that I would overcome ME/
CFS fairly, quickly with a lot of sleep and bedrest. I soon learned however,
that I had absolutely no understanding of how deeply this disease would
challenge me at my physical, cognitive and spiritual levels of being. I
watched myself go from a very active and high energy person to one who
could barely get out of bed, from a once optimistic person to one who could
barely see any light at the end of the tunnel and from a fairly understanding
person to one who struggled to be civil with others. ME/CFS was so grueling that I came to no longer know the person who I once was nor, what my
future might hold for me.

My journey through the research literature has helped me to understand
that my numerous, varied, persistent and debilitating physical, cognitive
and spiritual challenges, my co-existing medical conditions, my increased
mood disorders, and my more prolonged and continuous illness were not

uncommon for patients experiencing a more moderate to severe disease state. The literature also helped me to understand my experiences with the various treatment approaches and my "broader" experiences with the other possible patient outcomes. In many respects, my journey through the research literature helped me to appreciate that I was living with a chronic, invisible, debilitating, complex, multi-system disease that has many socio-cultural and economic challenges as well. ME/CFS, unlike any previous life experience, asked me to dig really, deep and find the strength within.

As I look back over my journey with ME/CFS, both in terms of my disease experiences and the research literature, there are a number of more "salient" moments that caused me to pause and reflect deeply on them. In this chapter, I would like to share some of these reflections. First, in terms of the research findings and secondly, in terms of living with a chronic, invisible and debilitating disease. Finally, I would like to share my reflections on how I drew meaning from my ME/CFS experiences and moved forward with my "new" life.

Reflections on the research literature

In terms of some of the more "salient" aspects of the research literature, I was first struck by the sizeable magnitude of this disease. Worldwide, an estimated 17 million individuals have been diagnosed with ME/CFS, or almost half of the entire Canadian population. This is a fairly, substantial number however, estimates suggest that 84-91% of all ME/CFS patients remain undiagnosed. Moreover, this disease touches not only the lives of the patients but so too, their loved ones, caregivers, employers, medical and research communities, and economies at large. In fact, the overall cost burden of ME/CFS, per annum, is an estimated $24 billion to the U.S. economy while, the costs of this disease to families, caregivers, employers and the U.S. society at large, are an estimated $18-51 billion. The personal, social and economic impacts of this disease ripple throughout many levels of our society, potentially touching the lives of many people who we know and love.

I was also struck by the fact that ME/CFS is not a new phenomenon. In fact, it has been causing suffering since the 1850's and yet, there remains no known cause for this disease, no known underlying medical condition that explains it, no known lab test that can confirm it, no generally accepted biomarkers or medical scan that can diagnose it, no known treatment that results in a cure and the rendering of a diagnosis can be lengthy, sometimes taking up to 5 years. As a result of these factors, it is understandable why ME/CFS can be overlooked, misunderstood, judged, misdiagnosed and mistreated. All the while, patients are often left to struggle alone.

What we do know about ME/CFS however, is that it is a "serious, chronic, complex, multi-system disease" [1] that causes "dysfunction of the neurological, immune, endocrine and energy/metabolism systems" [2]. Moreover, nine symptom categories, that speak to this multi-system disease and the dysfunction that it can cause, have been identified. The five core symptom categories, or the symptoms that are more universally present and more severe in patients' disease experiences, are impaired day-to-day functioning due to the debilitating fatigue, post exertional malaise (PEM), sleep dysfunction, cognitive impairments and orthostatic intolerance (OI). Patients can also experience the four secondary symptom categories of pain, infection, immune problems and neuroendocrine manifestations. The possible accumulation of symptoms from each of these nine symptom categories, all acting in tandem, to varying degrees, add to the challenges, complexity and burden of living with this multi-system disease.

To complicate the patients' disease state further, co-existing medical conditions such as mood disorders, fibromyalgia (FMS), temporomandibular joint pain (TMJ), multiple chemical sensitivities (MCS) and irritable bowel syndrome (IBS) can all accompany ME/CFS. These co-existing disorders present with their own varied, relentless and debilitating symptoms. The potential accumulation of symptoms from each of the nine symptom categories plus, those of the co-existing medical disorders, all operating in tandem, only compound the challenges, devastation, complexities and burden of living with ME/CFS.

Patients' experiences with ME/CFS vary significantly, depending on the number, type, severity and duration of their symptoms. Individuals who experience a milder case of this disease are more likely to return to their former health levels fairly, quickly after disease onset while, individuals who experience a more moderate to severe case, may never recover. Some patients will experience ME/CFS for a short period of time, others for a prolonged and continuous period of time and yet others, will experience returning episodes of ME/CFS for periods of 6 months or longer, with relapses occurring many years later. Generally speaking, the patients' recovery rates are between 3 to 7 years, with some patients feeling better within 6 months and others, continuing to be ill 20 years later. Prognoses for a full recovery are generally, poor in adults and range from 0-12%. The variations in the disease's symptoms, severity and duration, and the degree of patient recovery, may only add to the misunderstandings and misconceptions about this disease. These variations may lead "others" to believe for example, that ME/CFS is mild, of a limited duration, inconsequential and with an expected full recovery.

As discussed throughout this book, the majority of ME/CFS patients' experiences are to the contrary. ME/CFS can be an extremely debilitating, long lasting and life changing illness, with a poor prognosis in adults. This disease can leave once vibrant and energetic individuals so debilitated that they are unable to function and fully participate in their daily lives. In fact, this disease leaves an estimated 25% of all patients immobilized and dependent on others for their daily care. In its more moderate to severe disease state, ME/CFS can totally consume patients' lives! In addition to the many physical, cognitive and spiritual challenges imposed by ME/CFS, many patients face severe lifestyle restrictions, social isolation, a loss of productivity, income and employment, increased work absences, higher medical costs, stigmatization, a lack of family, social and medical support, a crisis of identity, and quality of life and longevity concerns. In effect, patients can lose much of what they hold dear including, their hopes and dreams.

While the magnitude and impacts of ME/CFS are sizeable and far reaching, "others'" lack of awareness of and misconceptions about this disease are concerning and problematic. It is not uncommon for "others" to question for example, if ME/CFS is real, if patients are malingering and whether ME/CFS is "all in the patient's head". "Others'" misconceptions and judgements about this disease can leave patients feeling misunderstood, judged, alone, stigmatized and ashamed, further adding to the psychological upheaval, stress and burden of living with this disease. ME/CFS can relentlessly challenge patients on their physical, cognitive and spiritual levels of being and can leave much devastation in its wake – personally, socially and economically. Figure

8 provides a graphic depiction of the complexity of the ME/CFS disease state and its devastating effects on patients' lives.

Figure 8: A graphic depiction of the complexity of the ME/ CFS disease state and its effects on patients' lives

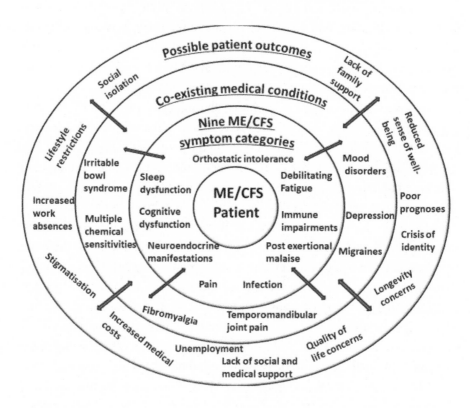

Research advances are critical to enhancing the social understanding of this disease, to advancing diagnostics and to identifying effective treatment options. Unfortunately, the research funding for ME/CFS is believed to be facing a "massive shortfall" [3]. In fact, an estimated 25-fold increase in annual funding is believed necessary, to be commensurate with ME/CFS' disease burden (i.e., number of people affected by an illness and the associated disability and early death rates). Much remains to be done! With enhanced funding and ongoing research however, patients can expect that, in time, there will be a better social understanding of ME/CFS, more support for patients, more effective diagnostic and treatment strategies, and a cure for this devastating disease.

In addition to these more "salient" aspects of the research literature, some of the research holds deep, personal meaning for me as well. First, the term ME/CFS, while it may sound rather benign is anything but. In my experience, the mention of a diagnosis of "chronic fatigue" was often met with misunderstanding, dismissiveness and judgement. I understand, we live in a society of incessant demands and little downtime. Fatigue can be a natural consequence of this lifestyle. However, the fatigue associated with ME/CFS is a pathophysiological exhaustion that can severely reduce one's ability to function and fully participate in his/her work, home, family and social life. So much remains to be done to help others understand that ME/CFS is not simply a variation of everyday fatigue but rather, is a fatigue that is situated at the far end of the fatigue spectrum – extreme exhaustion accompanied by severe physical, cognitive and spiritual impairments. Secondly, the "road map" that I was able to extrapolate from the literature spoke to my many physical, cognitive and spiritual challenges and in many respects, provided me with a real sense of comfort. To know that I was not alone in my disease experiences and that others had walked a similar path to mine was a relief – I was somehow, still within a norm! Third, the disease spectrum is fairly, broad and the severity and duration of the patients' disease state can make all the difference in their ME/CFS experiences and recovery. Fourth, a diagnosis can be a long and difficult journey, leaving many patients with no explanation for their illness nor their incessant struggles, sometimes for a very, long period of time. Fifth, ME/CFS is a complex, multi-system disease with no known cause or cure, and treatments need to be individualized, varying according to the individuals' unique responses and biological needs. Finally, the broader socio-cultural and economic impacts of ME/CFS can be equally challenging and burdensome.

The research literature has helped me on so many levels. I began for example, to deeply appreciate that I was not responsible for the onset of this disease, my lengthy diagnosis, my numerous and varied symptoms, my long recovery period, my difficulties in taking certain medications and my inability to participate in a graded exercise treatment (GET) program. Moreover, I began to relax and not be so hard on myself for having ME/CFS and my more severe experiences with it. The literature also enabled me to release myself from questioning why and comparing my experiences with those of other individuals who reported less symptom severity and recovered within a short period of time. Ultimately, the research helped me to respect my experiences with this disease and to not accept other people's misconceptions, judgements and opinions about me or this disease. I now, quietly accept and honor my truth. Finally, I have learned to trust in my body's wisdom – it will guide me through this disease including, the treatment approaches that best address my own, individual needs. In many respects, the research has helped me to better deal with this disease – mind, body and soul, and to embrace my life again. The research findings have been comforting and liberating, and have been a very, important part of my healing process.

Reflections on living with a chronic, invisible and debilitating disease

Over the years, I have found myself thinking deeply about living with a chronic, invisible and debilitating disease. From my point of view, it is often only when we experience such illnesses ourselves, that we begin to really think about and truly, appreciate what individuals who suffer from them go through every day. As a result of my journey with ME/CFS, I have come to understand that chronic and invisible diseases come in many forms and can affect anyone, at any point in time, for any number of reasons. Moreover, these diseases while not always life threatening, can threaten many aspects of the individual's life, leaving him/her to struggle with a new and demanding reality. A reality that he/she, like me, likely never conceived of as even being a possibility. Moreover, the impact that these diseases can have on our loved ones and the changes that can occur in our relationships with friends and colleagues, can also be sources of pain and loss. Chronic, invisible and debilitating diseases can insidiously alter so many aspects of a patient's life.

Admittedly, we all struggle, to varying degrees, with aspects of our daily lives but, a chronic, invisible and debilitating disease can make those struggles all the more difficult. As I have come to learn, these diseases can take a great deal of fortitude and courage to get up each day and face the relentless physical, cognitive and spiritual challenges of a disease. Simple things that we so often take for granted like standing without effort, walking and breathing without difficulty, thinking without cognitive exhaustion and living without constant psychological upheaval, can all change very quickly. Chronic and invisible diseases, while not apparent to an onlooker, can be relentless and can make the simplest of life's demands arduous and overwhelming for the individuals who live with them.

The multitude of losses that can accompany these diseases can, at times, also be unbearable. In my case, I faced the loss of my physical and cognitive abilities, my sense of connectedness and spiritual well-being, my high energy levels, my stamina and athleticism, my career, my ability to socialize and travel, my sense of adventure, joy and gratitude, my ability to dream and achieve new heights, my optimism and self-confidence and sadly, some friends. In many respects, I felt like I had lost essential parts of myself, as though my "essence" was in crisis. These losses cut me deeply and left me disillusioned, angry, sad and in despair. Perhaps, it was the accumulation of all of these losses at once or perhaps, it was feeling like a bystander in my own life and having very little energy to do anything about it or perhaps, it was my inability to get back up and get back to my life through my usual determination, will power and optimism but, ME/CFS stripped away fundamental parts of me. Parts of myself that I never, ever thought I could lose and as hard as I tried, I could not get back to the life that I once embraced, the life that once filled me with joy, gratitude and a sense of purpose. The life that in many respects, I had sculpted for myself. These losses had a profound effect on me! So many losses that remained invisible to "others".

This chronic, invisible and debilitating disease was so life limiting and life changing that I began to struggle with who I once was, who I was becoming and what might ultimately, lie before me. To remain sane, I had no choice but to revisit some of my life's assumptions and "world views". I had for example, always assumed that I would have good health, be able to set new goals and achieve new heights, be cognitively adept, have a career that I loved, have an active social life, and be able to fully embrace and live my life. I had also naively, assumed that nothing except my own self limitations would change that. As a result of this illness experience however, I have had to reexamine these assumptions and adjust my "world views" accordingly. In order to come to terms with my "new" physical, cognitive and spiritual reality, I had to let go of who I once believed I was, how I saw myself in the world and some of my long-held dreams and aspirations. Essentially, I had to peel away some of my "former" ways of viewing my world, to make room for my "new" life and my acceptance of that "new" life. This was not an easy process and I often felt like I was going back to the drawing board of my entire life, to make sense of it and to rescript it. However, the life that I was having to rescript, according to my "new" life's realities, was a life that I was not sure that I wanted to embrace. Compared to the life that I once lived, this "new" life seemed broken and so limited. As a result of this chronic, invisible and debilitating disease, I struggled profoundly to make sense of my "new" life and chart a "new" course.

All this to say, moving forward, I hope to be more mindful of the many struggles that can accompany individuals' chronic, invisible and debilitating disease experiences, to extend more kindness and compassion towards them, and to be less judgmental of them and their circumstances. While I may not visibly see or definitively know what these individuals are going through, their illness and all its inherent challenges are real and profoundly life altering. In watching the movie "The Shack", with Sam Worthington and Octavia Spencer (2017), I was moved by the following words which I believe, are pertinent to this discussion – "with every act of kindness, the universe changes, and nothing is ever the same again". Such powerful words for me to move forward with and to extend both to others and to myself.

Reflections on how I drew meaning from my ME/CFS experiences and moved forward with my "new" life

Over the years, I have found myself reflecting on how I might draw meaning from my ME/CFS experiences, what changes I might make to contribute to my overall sense of physical, cognitive and spiritual well-being, and how I might cobble together a life that was, once again, joyful and meaningful to me. In the remainder of this chapter, I would like to share these reflections.

As with many life changing events, a challenging and debilitating disease can be an important conduit for transformational change. My journey with ME/CFS has certainly provided me with opportunities to transform my heart and mind – to change my ways of feeling and thinking about my world. In struggling with my high levels of fatigue and having insufficient energy to get me through my days for example, I began to realize, at a more fundamental level than ever before, just how taxing and detrimental negative energy was to my mind, body and soul. My own and other people's negative thoughts, gossip or judgements could really weigh me down and could instantaneously, drain the little energy that I did have, leaving me even more exhausted, irritable, impatient and struggling all the more to cope with my daily life. Interestingly, during the initial years of this illness, I would also repeatedly hear a refrain of Buddha's words in my thoughts as follows – "speak only endearing speech, speech that is welcomed. Speech, when it brings no evil to others is a pleasant thing" (Buddha). As a result of these experiences, I have become more vigilant about wanting to hear about the good things in people's lives, positively reframing my negative thoughts and accepting that it is ok for me to walk away from or limit my time with negative people and situations. I am also cognizant, more than ever before, of the fact that I choose at every given moment of my life to be negative, judgmental and gossipy or positive, open and uplifting. It is within my power to change my attitude and my behaviors! Honoring my health needs, reframing my negative thoughts, seeking out more positive interactions and finding things, no matter how small or simple, that bring joy to my life and a smile to my face, every day, have been welcome changes in my life. Changes that have brought me a greater sense of happiness, peace and well-being.

My journey with ME/CFS has also afforded me opportunities to re-visit and release some of my former behaviors. Behaviors that were no longer serving my well-being. Prior to ME/CFS for example, I was a doer and jumped into things whether it was helping someone or doing something that perhaps, no one else wanted to do or had the time for but, needed to be done (at least from my perspective). With ME/CFS however, expending my limited energy to help someone or do something, really cost me. In many respects, I no longer had the energy to do, think or be the person who I most wanted to be so, I had to seriously consider where I was going to expend my very, limited energy. To do otherwise, caused me to relapse really, badly and struggle deeply. As a result of my reflections on this particular disease experience, I now accept that just because no one else raises his/her hand to help someone or do something, does not mean that I, as a doer, need to assume that responsibility. Besides, not everything needs to be done at this very moment and perhaps, it may not need to be done at all. People's wants and desires can be limitless! I now find myself thinking more deeply about my involvement in a situation, deciding if I can or want to help, whether that action is indeed necessary and whether that action is conducive to my overall well-being. Discerning what is essential verses "nice to do" has been critical to my overall health and sense of well-being! I have also come to the realize that there will always be a perceived need whether my own, other individuals' or life's situations but, giving to the point of having nothing left to give, profits no one. In fact, such giving can be soul diminishing rather than life giving, for all concerned. More than ever before, I now find myself attentively listening to my body and respecting its needs, discerning whether I can help others (rather than just jumping into the situation without question) and trying to live as normal a life as possible, without putting myself into the "push-crash" cycle of over-exertion and relapse. I believe that all these approaches are more thoughtful, better balance life's demands with my own self-care and are an important part of my physical, cognitive and spiritual well-being.

This disease experience has also made me more conscious of the fact that, while we may set goals and identify a path that we would like to walk in life, anything can happen, at any point in time along the way. We do not always get to choose "what" happens to us or "when" it may occur. I now more deeply appreciate that our life experiences, which may come gift wrapped in many forms including that of disease, can be incredible learning opportunities. While I was, admittedly, not enamored with the "what" and "when" of this particular life experience, I now understand that I do get to choose how I think and feel about it, and what I will take away from it. I also realize and accept that no matter what I face each day nor how challenging my life might get, it is up to me to decide whether I will rise from the "ashes" of this disease experience a little kinder, more courageous, wiser and loving, or whether I will allow this experience to break my spirit, leaving me negative, angry, bitter and resentful. From my perspective, it is my choice as to whether I react or respond to this experience and the "lessons" that I choose to draw from it that will make the difference in my life. If I approach this experience for what I now believe it is, a learning, healing and liberating opportunity, with an open mind and heart, courage and seeking God's guidance (Buddha, the Great Spirit, Yahweh, Mohammed, the universal energy force, the enlightened energy or whatever one's particular belief or view), I can grow from it and hopefully, be a little more open, compassionate and loving towards others and life itself.

I have also discovered that there may be times in life, such as a profound illness and loss, when no amount of determination, positive thinking or will power, is sufficient to overcome the circumstances. There were many times, throughout my life, when I accomplished things on the basis of my sheer will power and positive thinking but, with this particular life experience, I could not positive think nor will myself back to health, no matter how hard I tried. It was as though these abilities had been severely compromised and perhaps, even lost to me as well. I often pondered if this illness was so insidious that nothing about my usual modus operandi could overcome it. As I continued to reflect on this situation, I wondered whether there may be times in life when a life experience hits us so hard that we are thrown off balance, off of our body's "natural" equilibrium. Essentially, rendering our usual modus operandi ineffective. Akin to entering a vortex and being tossed about, with little opportunity to make sense of what is happening and "ground" ourselves. Perhaps, it is only with time and through the process of understanding, adapting, adjusting and accepting our "new" reality – our "new" equilibrium, that our characteristic traits of determination, positive thinking and will power start to reappear again.

I do not have the answer to this but, I do believe that this was a part of my journey and healing process.

This illness experience has further served to reemphasize that the lens that I use to look at a given situation affects what I see, what I feel, what I think and ultimately, what action I will take. By changing the angle and focus of my lens, I can change my perspective and in so doing, my attitude. Ultimately, it is again my choice as to whether this experience or life's experiences in general, are positive, negative, abundant or lacking. As William James aptly wrote, "people can alter their lives by altering their attitudes". Admittedly, this is not always an easy task when one is facing a chronic and debilitating illness, as the challenges can be relentless, the pain wearing and the sorrows deep. In recognizing and accepting my responsibility for changing my lens, my perspective and ultimately, my attitude towards this experience, I now look at my life and my circumstances a little more positively. I now try for example, to be more patient with and to not get down on myself when relapses occur. I also attempt to see these relapses as temporary setbacks and look to my tomorrows, as better days to come.

Consciously choosing a healthy lifestyle and doing what one can to be healthy, as I have learned, are not always a guarantee of a healthy outcome. Throughout my life, I was conscious of making healthy choices and living a fairly, healthy lifestyle. When I received my ME/CFS diagnosis I was, therefore, perplexed as to why I had this debilitating disease. My journey through the research literature however, helped me to understand and accept that there is no known cause or scientific explanation for this disease. In fact, there are varied and numerous causes, some of which are genetic, viral, immune, neurological or possibility, a combination of any number of factors working together. Factors that are not entirely, within an individual's control. A disease can thus, seemingly befall individuals for any number of reasons. None the less, this illness was humbling, for as much as I thought that I was in control of my health, for no obvious reason, this illness took center stage of my life. The unintended entered my life. Whether it be happenstance, synchronicity, karma, destiny or a combination thereof, the unintended drastically changed my life, in ways that I could never have imagined.

While I have always enjoyed the more "positive" outcomes of happenstance, synchronicity, karma or destiny, I have been more reticent to embrace the more "negative" outcomes. I have however, through this experience, come to more deeply appreciate that whatever the outcome, maybe it is life unfolding in a manner that will ultimately, be more life enriching for me. I think here of the dissolution of a marriage. At the time of the marital breakup, there can be a great deal of sadness and questioning of where to from here. As time passes though, we may have an opportunity to meet a life partner with whom we share a more loving and meaningful relationship. The initial sadness and bleakness that surrounded the marital breakup ultimately, had a more positive outcome. An outcome that may not have happened otherwise. Similarly, a rainbow often follows the darkest and harshest of rainstorms – emerging and filling the sky with light and a beautiful spectrum of colors. A period of uncertainty and darkness is again, followed by light and beauty. I also think here of my dad and the short time that I had with him following his cancer diagnosis. During that time of deep sorrow, I was able to sit and talk with my dad heart to heart. I came to see him as never before for his courage, integrity, faith, love of family and deep respect for life. I also came to more deeply, appreciate my dad for his strength of character and the very loving and important role that he played in my life. This was such a heart wrenching time and yet, a time that was filled with many moments of love, deep connection and new understandings. All this to say, out of some of the most difficult and darkest of times, there can also be light, beauty, self-understanding and life enriching experiences. I would add, given my particular perspective on life that sometimes, it may only be with the passage of time that we come to see, understand and appreciate God's guiding hand in our life (or whatever one's particular belief or view).

Accepting that I had ME/CFS took me quite a while. It took me even longer to accept that my life was radically changed, and that maybe, just maybe, my health status was as good as it was going to get. Over the first couple of years following my diagnosis, I frequently told my doctors that I would overcome this disorder and regain my health and the way of life that I had so much enjoyed. Then one day, my psychologist asked me – "Deb, what if this is as good as it gets"? I remember sitting there in utter astonishment thinking, "how can that be? I just need a bit more time. I will push through this and get my life back". At that exact moment, I recalled my GP's words "at some point Deb, you may have to accept that this is now your life and make the most of it". Their words, which I was finally able to acknowledge, seemed like such a cruel reality. To contemplate the rest of my life as resting, resting, resting, feeling ill, being in pain and being too tired to live my life fully and passionately, was inconceivable. I was still so determined to live life on my terms. I realized though, that there was a wisdom in their counsel and that it was perhaps time to turn the page and consider this possibility, to consider accepting what was increasingly apparent – my "new reality" – my "new norm" – my "new life".

The idea that my life might continue to be so limited and that I needed to "accept it", seemed incomprehensible. It was as though accepting this disease meant giving up the hope that I would one day overcome it and return to the life that I loved. I struggled to find my fulcrum – that balance point between embracing acceptance and yet, continuing to hold out hope for a better health outcome. This "dichotomy" or cognitive dissonance created such a tension in me, for the longest time. I have now reached a point however, where I accept that my health status may be as good as it is going to get and that I need to live my best life. However, the determined person that I am (some may call it stubborn), continues to hold out hope for recovery. Hope continues to burn like a candle in my darkest of days and nights, comforting and allowing me to believe that all things remain possible. Hope has been my best friend in my greatest hours of need. My faith also grounds me from the shifting sands of this disease, my love for my family, friends and life itself fills me with joy, and my gratitude for my life continues to inspire and fill me with promise. Without hope, faith, love and gratitude, I do not know what I would have done nor, where I would be at this very moment. While I remain uncertain as to what my ultimate health outcome will be, I am confident that whatever it is, it will be positive and will serve my higher good. Perhaps, this is acceptance in its ultimate form.

I have been extremely fortunate throughout my ME/CFS journey as I have had excellent medical support. Both of my doctors understood that having a chronic, invisible and debilitating disease can be challenging and life changing. Throughout the years, they have offered me their understanding, compassion and excellent medical advice. They have been a place of solace, validation and encouragement for me. In many respects, as mentioned earlier, they watered my parched soul. Gratefully, my GP also encouraged me to trust in my body's wisdom, allowing it to guide me through the different treatment approaches. When my body rebuked some of the medications and was extremely sensitive to exercise therapy for example, she recommended that I heed my body's wisdom and cease the medications and therapy, immediately. Both of my doctors have treated me with respect, understood that I was not malingering and stood by me, throughout all these years. On the basis of my experiences, I would highly recommend that patients find compassionate, supportive and knowledgeable doctors, as they will be precious gifts throughout ones ME/CFS journey.

Moreover, for those individuals who can continue to work during their illness, I hope that you have an understanding and compassionate manager. A manager who will work with you to meet both your work and health demands. As we saw in the research literature, nearly two thirds of all ME/CFS patients are limited in their ability to work, with less than 35% working on a full-time basis and 40% on a part time basis [4]. I can certainly, attest to the importance of having an understanding and compassionate manager. When I was suffering with chronic vertigo, I was very, fortunate as my senior managers allowed me to work from home 1-2 days a week. This flexibility allowed me to meet both my work and health requirements. I will be forever grateful to these individuals – their kindness and compassion are indelibly marked on my heart.

At one point along my journey, I also realized that I needed to stop dwelling on the challenges, losses and disappointments of this disease. I needed to take back my power and accept my "new" reality, make the most of my "new" life and tap the depths of my spiritual connectedness. When all I saw were my struggles and losses, my outlook on life could be really, bleak leaving me to struggle even more. While I recognized that it was healthy to acknowledge my struggles, despair and losses, I also knew that if I was going to "lighten my load", I needed to try to see my life in a more positive light. I was after all, fortunate as this disease is typically not life threatening and I was still fairly, physically mobile. Initially, by simply telling myself and eventually, believing that I was going to be ok, no matter what my health outcome was, I would be filled with a sense of promise. By giving thanks for my life, even though it was a small semblance of what it once was, I would feel more grounded and could once again, feel the warmth of God's love (or whatever one's, particular belief or view). Moreover, I recognized that I needed to live my life more "mindfully" and tap the depths of my spiritual connectedness – that deep place within me, whether it be faith, strength of character or life's own sustaining force. When I focused solely on my struggles and losses, I lost touch with my deep place of inner knowing, that place of trusting that all is well in my world, that place that uplifts my soul, that place that fills me with hope, joy and gratitude.

ME/CFS required me to dig deep, to a deeper part of myself, to a belief and trust in life itself. To trusting that God (or whatever one's belief or view) holds me in his/her hands, knows where I am going and what I need to experience to get there. Perhaps, it is through this disease experience that I will ultimately, fulfill my potential as a physical and spiritual being. I do not know my health outcome and I do not know the purpose for all of this, all I know is that when I enter that place of connectedness, that deep place of inner knowing, there is no question that all is and will continue to be well in my life. Admittedly, this realization took me some time.

While I may never fully understand why this disease and it many challenges continue to be a part of my life, I fundamentally believe that this experience holds deep meaning and valuable life lessons for me. As a friend aptly suggested to me one day, "God works in mysterious ways". On my part, I need to have faith that my higher good is being served. While this disease state is certainly, not what I would have chosen for my life, it may be what I need to live a more fulfilled and enriching life. I have long believed that life is eternal and that we operate in both the physical and spiritual realms – that ultimately, both realms are one. The physical realm and my experiences in it can help with my spiritual development. Conversely, my spiritual development can help me live a more conscious and loving existence in the physical realm. Perhaps, it is through circumstances such as disease and loss, that we open ourselves up to living more consciously in both realms, and to trusting that a higher purpose is indeed being served. To trusting that no matter what my life's circumstances, my life has value, purpose and is rich with possibilities.

In many respects, this illness has been a journey back to a more abundant inner life. It has been an opportunity to look inward, to self-love and self-nurturing, to reawakening my soul, to gratitude for my life and my God, and to accepting that ultimately, there is a season and reason for all things. I do not always need to understand the reason for everything, I just need to keep trying to do my best and live my best life, trusting in life and its goodness. This experience has also made me more conscious of my need to embrace my "new" normal, live more in the moment, make the most of each day and live one day at a time. I am also, more mindfully aware of the goodness that surrounds me. I cherish my time, more than ever before, with my family and friends. I cannot explain the joy that I feel when I hear the laughter of my great nephews and nieces, the pleasure I get from watching birds play in a bird bath, the love I feel for Brodi when I watch her enjoy her life or the excitement and gratitude that I have for life, its beauty and its abundance. I am further learning to surrender some of my long-held dreams, to make room for new ones. Perhaps, as Joseph Campbell wrote, life is about "let(ting) go of the life we planned, so as to accept the one that is waiting for us". Perhaps, it is life's wisdom that will help me discern when I need to push through in my doing and achieving of things, to being and accepting that life may be asking me to travel a different road from the one that I am on. A road that is filled with an abundance and richness that I may never have conceived of and to a life that may have beckoned me all along.

Maybe, I needed to experience the loss of my life as I knew it, so that I could open-up more to life as it is. The past is over, the future is not known but the present is rich with opportunity. As Buddha aptly wrote "be where you are; otherwise you will lose your life". This disease experience has shown me that I need to focus on what I do have, to be conscious of the fact that my life is bountifully blessed and to be grateful. It has further shown me that I need to remain present to my life's daily blessings, letting them fill me with joy, well-being and a sense of abundance.

Admittedly, with all the turmoil of the physical, cognitive and spiritual challenges of this disease, I lost my true north. I lost my sense of who I was, both as a physical and a spiritual being. I have for so long, believed that life is a privilege and I have sought to live mine as fully as possible. I do not want to simply survive, I want to thrive! While this disease and its many challenges continue to be a part of my life, I appreciate more deeply than ever before, that life is a very precious gift – I am alive, I am loved, and I am very blessed. I am here, I am now, and I am in this precious and beautiful moment. I have an opportunity each day to start anew, see anew, think anew, be anew and live anew. Every moment of every day, I have an opportunity to express a new idea, to touch and be touched by someone or something that moves me, to feel joy, to be inspired, to rejoice, to love, to be loved and to be kind. Life itself beckons me to believe in its possibilities, to live fully and to rejoice and embrace it, whatever my circumstances. Ultimately, life's preciousness, richness and beauty have become all-the-more poignant.

In summary, my journey with ME/CFS has invited me to reflect on some of the more "salient" points of the research literature and on my lived experiences with this chronic, invisible and debilitating disease. It has also invited me to look deep within, to sift through my life, to question some of my world views, to surrender some of my long-held dreams to make room for new ones, to embrace my life's many blessings and to be grateful. In many respects, ME/CFS has asked me to dig deep and to find the strength within. As a result, I have been able to move more confidently and joyfully forward with my "new" life.

In concluding this book, it is my sincerest hope that I have provided you, the reader, with a road map to understanding ME/CFS and that you now, have a deeper appreciation of this disease – its far reaching impacts, what it is, how it manifests itself, how it differs amongst patients, its risk factors and possible causes, its relentless challenges and debilitating effects and finally, its varied patient outcomes, prognoses and treatments. It is my further hope that in sharing my personal journey with a more moderate to severe disease experience, that some light has been shed on how the numerous, varied and relentless physical, cognitive and spiritual challenges can devastate patients' lives. Finally, it is my hope that my ME/CFS experiences and journey through the research literature have, in some small way, touched the hearts and minds of patients, their loved ones, employers, colleagues and medical professionals alike, and that this book has served to reduce some of the misconceptions and misunderstandings surrounding this disease and the people who struggle with it. It is my deepest hope however, that individuals living with this disease and their loved ones, feel less alone and have found some comfort and hope in the pages of this book.

In parting, I would like to leave you with the following Irish blessing:

May your joys be as bright as the morning, and your sorrows merely be shadows that fade in the sunlight of love. May you have enough happiness to keep you sweet, enough trials to keep you strong, enough sorrow to keep you human, enough hope to keep you happy, enough failure to keep you humble, enough success to keep you eager, enough friends to give you comfort, enough faith and courage in yourself to banish sadness, enough wealth to meet your needs and one thing more, enough determination to make each day a more wonderful day than the one before.

My warm and many blessings to you.

Notes

Preface

1. IACFS/ME (International Association for ME/CFS) (2012). *ME/CFS: A primer for clinical practitioners.* Chicago, IL: IACFS/ME.
2. The Lancet (2015). What's in a name? Systemic exertion intolerance disease. *The Lancet*, February, 385(9969):663.

Chapter 1

1. Public Health Agency of Canada (2013). Chronic diseases. https:// cbpp-pcpe.phac-aspc.gc.ca/chronic-diseases/.
2. IDA (Invisible Disabilities Association) (2019, p. 1). Invisible disability. https://invisibledisabilities.org/what-is-an-invisible-disability/.
3. ME Action (2019, p. 1). What is ME/CFS. https://www.meaction.net/ about/what-is-me/. (accessed 2019-05-19).
4. CDC (Centers for disease control and prevention) (2019). What is ME/CFS. https://www.cdc.gov/me-cfs/about/index.html. (accessed 19-05-2019).
5. Mayo Clinic (2019). ME/CFS symptoms and causes. https://www. mayoclinic.org/diseases-conditions/chronic-fatigue-syndrome/symptoms-causes/syc-20360490. (accessed 19-05-2019).
6. Valdez, A., E. Hancock, S. Adebayo, D. Kiernicki, D. Proskauer, J. Attewell, L. Bateman, A. DeMaria, C. Lapp, P. Rowe & C. Proskauer (2019). Estimating prevalence, demographics, and costs of ME/CFS using large scale medical claims data and machine learning. *Frontiers in Pediatrics*, 2018, 6:412. Published online January 8, 2019. doi: 10.3389/fped.2018.00412.
7. CDC (Centers for disease control and prevention) (2014). Recognition and management of CFS: A resource guide for health care professionals. http://www.cdc.gov/cfs/toolkit. (accessed 3/10/2015).

8. Favaro, A. (2018). CFS in Canada even worse than we thought: Survey. www/ctv/news.ca/health/chr-fat-sym-in-canada-even-worse-than-we-thought-survey-1.3539595.

9. Callaway, E. (2011). CFS: Life after XMRV. http://www.nature.com/news/2011/110603/full/news. (accessed 3/10/2016).

10. Van't Leven, M., G. Zielhuis, J. Van Der Meer, A. Verbeek & G. Bleijenberg (2010). CFS vs. fatigue – Fatigue and CFS like complaints in the general population. *European Journal of Public Health,* 20(3):251-257.

11. Jason, L., S. Torres-Harding & M. Njoku (2006). The face of CFS in the U.S. CFIDS (Chronic fatigue and immune dysfunction syndrome). *Chronicle.* https://www.researchgate.net/publication/ 236995875The FaceofCFSintheUS.

12. Kraft, S. (2015). What is chronic fatigue syndrome? What causes chronic fatigue syndrome? *Medical News Today*, February 13, 2015. http://www.medicalnewstoday.com/articles/184802.

13. NIH (National Institute of Health) (2017). ME/CFS and Fibromyalgia Awareness Day, May 12, 2017. https://www. nih.gov/research-training/medical-research-initiatives/mecfs/me-cfs-fibromyalgia-international-awareness-day.

14. Carruthers, B. and M. van de Sande (2005). *ME/CFS: A clinical case definition and guidelines for medical practitioners: An overview of the Canadian Consensus Document.* Haworth Medical Press Inc., Canada.

15. Jason. L., C. Holbert, S. Torres-Harding & R. Taylor (2004). Stigma and the term CFS. *Journal of Disability Policy Studies,* 14(4):222-228.

16. Institute of Medicine of the National Academies: Committee on the diagnostic criteria for ME/CFS (2015). *Beyond ME/CFS: Redefining an illness.* Washington (DC): National Academies Press (US). February 2015.

17. Reynolds, K., S. Vernon, E. Bouchery & W. Reeves (2004). The economic impact of CFS. *Cost Effectiveness and Resource Allocation,* 2(4).

18. Jason, L. and J. Richman (2008). How science can stigmatize: The case of CFS. *Journal of CFS,* 14(4):85-103.

19. Jason, L., M. Benton, L. Valentine, A. Johnson & S. Torres-Harding (2008). The economic impact of ME/CFS: Individual and societal costs. *Dynamic Medicine,* 7(1).

20. 2020 Health (2017). Counting the cost of CFS/ME: Full Report. https://www.meassociation.org.uk/wp-content/uploads/2020Health-Counting-the-Cost-Sept-2017.pdf.

21. The Myalgic Encephalomyelitis Association of Ontario (2008). Easing the economic and social burden of a chronic condition: Addressing the ME/CFS epidemic. Recommendations to the Federal Minister of Health, 2/27/2008.

22. McGrath, S. (2018a). A new research landscape emerges in America. http://www:mecfsresearchreview.me/2018/04/26/a-new-research-landscape-emerges-in-america/.

23. Spotila, J. (2018). NIH funding for ME goes down in 2018. https://www.occupyme.net/2018/10/21/nih-funding-for-me-goes-down-in-2018/.

24. Radford, G. and S. Chowdhury (2016). ME/CFS research funding: An overview of activity by major institutional funders included on the dimensions database. https://www.meassociation.org.uk/wp-content/uploads/mecfs-research-funding-report-2016.pdf.

25. McGrath, S. (2018). There is a yawning gap in ME/CFS research funding: Take action. http://www:mecfsresearch.me/2018/05/08/ thereis-a-yawning-gap-in-me-cfs-research-funding-take-action.9)

26. Memorial University (2018). Team Grant: ME/CFS collaborative project (ME/CFS collaborative project). http://www:research-tools-mun.ca/funding/opportunites/team-grant-me-cfs-collaborative-project-myalgic-encephalomyelitis-chronic-fatigue-syndrome-collaborative-project/.

27. Canadian Press (2019). Federal agency announces $1.4 million to research chronic fatigue syndrome. https://montrealgazette.com/news/local-news/health-canada-announces-1-4-million-to-research-chronic-fatigue-syndrome.

28. Dimmock, M., M. Mirin & L. Jason (2016). Estimating the disease burden of ME/CFS in the United States and its relation to research funding. *Journal of Medical Therapy,* 1: DOI: 10.15761/JMT.1000102.

Chapter 2

1. Institute of Medicine of the National Academies: Committee on the diagnostic criteria for ME/CFS (2015). *Beyond ME/CFS: Redefining an illness.* Washington (DC): National Academies Press (US). February 2015.
2. NICE (National Institute for Healthcare Excellence) (2007). Chronic fatigue syndrome/myalgic encephalomyelitis (or encephalopathy): Diagnosis and management clinical guidelines. August 2007. https://www.nice.org.uk/guidance/cg53/resources/chronic-fatigue-syndromemyalgic-encephalomyelitis-or-encephalopathy-diagnosis-and-management-pdf-975505810885.
3. Carruthers, B., M. van de Sande, K. De Meirleir, N. Klimas, G. Broderick, T. Mitchell, D. Staines, A. Powles, N. Speight, R. Vallings, L. Bateman, B. Baumgarten-Austrheim, D. Bell, N. Carlo-Stella, J. Chia, A. Darragh, D. Jo, D. Lewis, A. Light, S. Marshall-Gradisbik, I. Mena, J. Mikovits, K. Miwa, M. Murovska, M. Pall & S. Stevens (2017). Myalgic encephalomyelitis: International Consensus Criteria. *Journal of Internal Medicine,* 282(4):353.
4. Kindlon, T. (2017). Treatment and management of CFS/ME: All roads lead to Rome. *Journal of Health Psychology*, 2(9):1146-1154.
5. Shukla, D. and K. Shukla (2016, p. 1). Spiritual health: Definition and applications in clinical care. *Journal, Indian Academy of Clinical Medicine,* 17(1):6-7. http://medind.nic.in/jac/t16/i1/jact16i1p6.pdf.
6. Ghaderi, A., S. Tabatabaei, S. Nedjat, M. Javadi & B. Larijani (2018). Explanatory definition of the concept of spiritual health: A qualitative study in Iran. *Journal of Medical Ethics and History of Medicine*, 11:3.

Chapter 3

1. New York Times Health (2009). Chronic Fatigue: In-depth report. The New York Times Health. http://www.nytimes.com/health/guides/disease/chronic-fatigue-syndrome. (accessed 3/10/15).
2. University of Maryland Medical System (2013). *Chronic Fatigue Syndrome: An in-depth report on the causes, diagnosis and treatment of CFS.* http://umm.edu/health/medical/reports/articles/chrnic-fatigue-syndrome/. (accessed 3-10-2015).

3. IDAC (Invisible Disabilities Association of Canada) (2012). Chronic Fatigue Syndrome/Myalgic Encephalomyelitis: Definition, diagnosis, symptoms and treatment. http://www.disabilityliving.ca/disability-canada-invisible-disabilities-association-resources/.

4. Institute of Medicine of the National Academies: Committee on the diagnostic criteria for ME/CFS (2015). *Beyond ME/CFS: Redefining an illness*. Washington (DC): National Academies Press (US). February 2015.

5. CDC (Centers for disease control and prevention) (2014). *Recognition and management of CFS: A resource guide for health care professionals*. http://www.cdc.gov/cfs/toolkit. (accessed 3/10/2015).

6. University of Maryland Medical System (2013, p. 1). *Chronic Fatigue Syndrome: An in-depth report on the causes, diagnosis and treatment of CFS*. http://umm.edu/health/medical/reports/articles/chrnic-fatigue-syndrome/. (accessed 3-11-2015).

7. Kraft, S. (2015). What is chronic fatigue syndrome? What causes chronic fatigue syndrome? *Medical News Today*, February 13, 2015. http://www.medicalnewstoday.com/articles/184802.

8. Wojcik, W., D. Armstrong & R. Kanaan (2011). CFS: Labels, meanings and consequences. *Journal of Psychosomatic Research,* 70(6):500-504.

9. Jason. L., C. Holbert, S. Torres-Harding & R. Taylor (2004). Stigma and the term CFS. *Journal of Disability Policy Studies,* 14(4):222-228.

10. Institute of Medicine of the National Academies: Committee on the diagnostic criteria for ME/CFS (2015, pp. 227-228). *Beyond ME/CFS: Redefining an illness*. Washington (DC): National Academies Press (US). February 2015.

11. The Lancet (2015). What's in a name? Systemic exertion intolerance disease. *The Lancet*, February, 385(9969):663.

12. IACFS/ME (International Association for ME/CFS) (2012). *ME/CFS: A primer for clinical practitioners*. Chicago, IL: IACFS/ME.

13. Institute of Medicine of the National Academies: Committee on the diagnostic criteria for ME/CFS (2015, p. 5). *Beyond ME/CFS: Redefining an illness*. Washington (DC): National Academies Press (US). February 2015.

14. Carruthers, B. and M. van de Sande (2005, p. 1). *ME/CFS: A clinical case definition and guidelines for medical practitioners: An overview of the Canadian Consensus Document.* Haworth Medical Press Inc., Canada.

15. Kraft, S. (2015, p. 1). What is chronic fatigue syndrome? What causes chronic fatigue syndrome? *Medical News Today,* February 13, 2015. http://www.medicalnewstoday.com/articles/184802.

16. 2020 Health (2017, p. 6). *Counting the cost of CFS/ME: Full Report.* https://www.meassociation.org.uk/wp-content/uploads/2020Health-Counting-the-Cost-Sept-2017.pdf.

17. ME Action (2019, p. 8). What is ME/CFS. https://www.meaction.net/about/what-is-me/. (accessed 05-19-2019).

18. Christley, Y., T. Duffy & C. Martin (2011, p. A31). Definitional criteria for chronic fatigue syndrome: A critical review. The *Journal of The International Society for Pharmacoeconomics and Outcomes Research,* 14(3):A31-A32.

19. Callaway, E. (2011). CFS: Life after XMRV. http://www.nature.com/news/2011/110603/full/news (accessed 3/10/2016).

20. CDC (Centers for disease control and prevention) (2012). Myalgic encephalomyelitis/chronic fatigue syndrome (ME/CFS). https://www.cdc.gov/me-cfs/index. (accessed 3/10/2015).

21. Seltzer, J. (2018, p. 1). Information for healthcare providers. https://me-pedia.org/wiki/info-for-healthcare-providers (July 29, 2018).

22. Brkic, S., S. Tomic, M. Ruzic & D. Maric (2011). Chronic Fatigue Syndrome. *Srpski Arhiv za Celokupno Lekarstvo,* 139(3-4):256.

23. Carruthers, B. and M. van de Sande (2005). *ME/CFS: A clinical case definition and guidelines for medical practitioners: An overview of the Canadian Consensus Document.* Haworth Medical Press Inc., Canada.

24. Mayo Clinic (2014). Diseases and conditions: Chronic fatigue syndrome. http://www.mayoclinic.org/diseases-conditions/chronicfatigue syndrome/basics. (accessed April 4, 2015).

25. Chu, L., I. Valencia, D. Garvert & J. Montoya (2018). Deconstructing post-exertional malaise in myalgic encephalomyelitis/chronic fatigue

syndrome: A patient-centered, cross-sectional survey. Plos One, 06-01-2018, https://doi.org/10.1371/journal.pone.0197811.

26. Canadian Institute of Health Research (2018). Working with patients and their families to improve health outcomes for people living with ME/CFS. cihr-irsc.gc.ca/e/51074.html.

27. Ortega-Hernandez, O. and Y. Shoenfeld (2009). Infection, Vaccination and Autoantibodies in CFS: Cause or coincidence? *Annals of the New York Academy of Sciences,* 1173:600(10).

28. Moss-Morriss, R., M. Spence & R. Hou (2011). The pathway from glandular fever to CFS: Can the cognitive behavioral model provide the map? *Psychological Medicine,* 41(5):1099-1107.

29. Kindlon, T. (2017). Treatment and management of CFS/ME: All roads lead to Rome. *Journal of Health Psychology,* 22(9):1146-1154.

30. Roberts, A., M. Charler, A. Papadopoulos, S. Wessely, T. Chalder & A. Cleare (2010). Does hypocortisolism predict a poor response to cognitive behavioraial therapy in CFS? *Psychological Medicine,* 40(3):515-522.

31. Arnett, S., L. Alleva, R. Korossy-Horwood & I. Clark (2011). CFS: A neuroimmunological model. *Medical Hypotheses,* 77(1):77-83.

32. Bai, N. (2011). Donor fatigue (restricting blood donations from persons with CFS). *Scientific American,* 305(1):26.

33. Lo, S-C., N. Pripuzova, B. Li, A. Komaroff, G-C. Hung & R. Wang (2010). Detection of MLV-related virus gene sequences in blood of patients with CFS and healthy blood donors. *Proceedings of the National Academy of Sciences of the USA,* 107(36):15874-15879.

34. Fletcher, M., X. Zeng, K. Maher, L. Levis, B. Hurwitz, M. Antoni, G. Broderick, N. Klimas & D. Unutmaz (2010). Biomarkers in CFS: Evaluation of natural killer cell function and dipeptidyl peptidase IV/CD26 (Biomarkers in CFS). *PLoS One,* 5(5):e.10817.

35. Nater, U., E. Maloney, C. Heim & W. Reeves (2011). Cumulative life stress in CFS. *Psychiatry Research,* 189(2):318-321.

36. Johnson, L., K. Schmaling, J. Dmochowski & D. Bernstein (2010). An investigation of victimization and the clinical course of chronic fatigue syndrome. *Journal of Health Psychology,* 15(3):351-361.

37. Arroll, M. (2013). Allostatic overload in ME/CFS. *Medical Hypotheses,* 81(3):506-508.

38. Besharat, M., A. Behpajooh, H. Poursharifi & F. Zarani (2011). Personality and CFS: The role of the five-factor model. *Asian Journal of Psychiatry*, 4(1):55-59.

39. Courjaret, J., C. Schotte, H. Wijnants, G. Moorkens & P. Cosyns (2009). CFS and DSM-IV personality disorders. *Journal of Psychosomatic Research,* 66(1):13-20.

40. Kempke, S., P. Luyten, S. Claes, P. Van Wambeke, P. Bekaert, L. Goossens & B. Van Houdenhove (2013). The prevalence and impact of early childhood trauma in ME/CFS patients. *Journal of psychiatric research*, 47(5):664-669.

41. Twisk, F. (2016). PACE: CBT and GET are not rehabilitative therapies. *The Lancet Psychiatry,* 3(2):PE6. http://doi.org/10.1016/S2215-0366(15)00554-4.

42. CFIDS (Chronic Fatigue and Immune Deficiency Syndrome) Association of America (2014). *CFS road to diagnosis survey*. Charlotte, NC: CFIDS Association of America.

43. NIH (National Institute of Health) (2017). ME/CFS and Fibromyalgia Awareness Day, May 12, 2017. https://www.nih.gov/research-training/medical-research-initiatives/mecfs/me-cfs-fibromyalgia-international-awareness-day.

44. Jason, L., S. Torres-Harding & M. Njoku (2006). The face of CFS in the U.S. CFIDS (Chronic fatigue and immune dysfunction syndrome). *Chronicle.* https://www.researchgate.net/publication/ 236995875TheFaceofCFSin theUS.

45. Park, J. and Gilmour H. (2017). *MUPS among adults in Canada: Comorbidity, health care use and employment.* Statistics Canada, catalogue no. 82-003-X, ISSN 1209-1367, Health Reports, Vol. 28, no. 3, pp. 3-8, March 2017.

46. Institute of Medicine of the National Academies: Committee on the diagnostic criteria for ME/CFS (2015, p. 73). *Beyond ME/CFS: Redefining an illness.* Washington (DC): National Academies Press (US). February 2015.

47. Carruthers, B., M. van de Sande, K. De Meirleir, N. Klimas, G. Broderick, T. Mitchell, D. Staines, A. Powles, N. Speight, R. Vallings & L. Bateman (2011). Myalgic encephalomyelitis: International Consensus Criteria. *Journal of Internal Medicine*, 282(4):327-338.

48. Jason, L., M. Sunnquist, A. Brown, M. Evans, S. Vernon, J. Furst & V. Simonis (2013). Examining case definition criteria for CFS and ME. *Fatigue: Biomedicine, Health & Behavior,* 2(1).

49. Jason, L., M. Evans, N. Porter, M. Brown, A. Brown, J. Hannell, V. Anderson, A. Lerch, K. De Meirleir & F. Friedberg (2010). The development of the revised Canadian ME/CFS case definition. *American Journal of Biochemistry and Biotechnology,* 6:120-135.

50. Carruthers, B., M. van de Sande, K. De Meirleir, N. Klimas, G. Broderick, T. Mitchell, D. Staines, A. Powles, N. Speight, R. Vallings, L. Bateman, B. Baumgarten-Austrheim, D. Bell, N. Carlo-Stella, J. Chia, A. Darragh, D. Jo, D. Lewis, A. Light, S. Marshall-Gradisbik, I. Mena, J. Mikovits, K. Miwa, M. Murovska, M. Pall & S. Stevens (2017). Myalgic encephalomyelitis: International Consensus Criteria. *Journal of Internal Medicine,* 282(4):353.

51. Institute of Medicine of the National Academies: Committee on the diagnostic criteria for ME/CFS (2015, p. 6). *Beyond ME/CFS: Redefining an illness*. Washington (DC): National Academies Press (US). February 2015.

52. Chu, L., I. Valencia, D. Garvert & J. Montoya (2019, p. 25). Onset patterns and course of ME/CFS. *Frontiers in Pediatrics*, February 5, 2019, https://doi.org/10.3389/fped.2019.00012.

53. Dellwo, A. (2014). TMJ in Fibromyalgia and Chronic fatigue syndrome: Is your jaw pain TMJ? December 15, 2014. www.questia.com.

54. Deary, V. and T. Chalder (2010). Personality and perfectionism in CFS: A closer look. *Psychology and Health,* 25(4):465-475.

55. Valero, S., N. Saez-Francas, N. Calvo, J. Alegre & M. Casas (2013). The role of neuroticism, perfectionism and depression in CFS: A structural equation modeling approach. *Comprehensive Psychiatry,* 54(7):1061-1067.

56. Maes, M. (2011). An intriguing and hitherto unexplained co-occurrence: Depression and chronic fatigue syndrome are manifestations of shared inflammatory, oxidative and nitrosative (IO & NS) pathways. *Progress in Neuropsychopharmacology and Biological Psychiatry*, 35(3):784-794.

57. Saez-Francas, N., S. Valero, N. Calvo, M. Goma-i-Freixanet, J. Alegre, T. de Sevilla & M. Casas (2014). CFS and personality: A case-control study using the alternative five factor model. *Psychiatry Research*, 216(3):373-378.

58. NICE (National Institute for Healthcare Excellence) (2007). Chronic fatigue syndrome/myalgic encephalomyelitis (or encephalopathy): Diagnosis and management clinical guidelines. August 2007. https://www.nice.org.uk/guidance/cg53/resources/chronic-fatigue-syndromemyalgic-encephalomyelitis-or-encephalopathy-diagnosis-and-management-pdf-975505810885.

59. CDC (Centers for disease control and prevention) (2012). https://me-pedia.org/wiki/Fukuda_criteria. (accessed 01-05-2018).

Chapter 4

1. IDA (Invisible Disabilities Association) (2017). How do you define invisible disability? https://invisible.disabilities.org/what-is-an-invisible-disability/.

2. University of Maryland Medical System (2013). *Chronic Fatigue Syndrome: An in-depth report on the causes, diagnosis and treatment of CFS*. http://umm.edu/health/medical/reports/articles/chrnic-fatigue-syndrome/. (accessed 3-10-2015).

3. Mayo Clinic (2019). ME/CFS symptoms and causes. https://www.mayoclinic.org/diseases-conditions/chronic-fatigue-syndrome/symptoms-causes/syc-20360490. (accessed 19-05-2019).

4. Institute of Medicine of the National Academies: Committee on the diagnostic criteria for ME/CFS (2015). *Beyond ME/CFS: Redefining an illness*. Washington (DC): National Academies Press (US). February 2015.

5. Seltzer, J. (2018). Information for healthcare providers. https://me-pedia.org/wiki/info-for-healthcare-providers (July 29, 2018).

6. ME Action (2019, p. 1). What is ME/CFS. https://www.meaction.net/about/what-is-me/. (accessed 05-19-2019).
7. The Lancet (2015). What's in a name? Systemic exertion intolerance disease. *The Lancet*, February, 385(9969):663.
8. Institute of Medicine of the National Academies: Committee on the diagnostic criteria for ME/CFS (2015, p. 77). *Beyond ME/CFS: Redefining an illness*. Washington (DC): National Academies Press (US). February 2015.
9. IACFS/ME (International Association for ME/CFS) (2012, p. 20). *ME/CFS: A primer for clinical practitioners*. Chicago, IL: IACFS/ME.
10. Carruthers, B. and M. van de Sande (2005, p. 12). *ME/CFS: A clinical case definition and guidelines for medical practitioners: An overview of the Canadian Consensus Document*. Haworth Medical Press Inc., Canada.
11. IDAC (Invisible Disabilities Association of Canada) (2012). Chronic Fatigue Syndrome/Myalgic Encephalomyelitis: Definition, diagnosis, symptoms and treatment. http://www.disabilityliving.ca/disability-canada-invisible-disabilities-association-resources/.
12. Jason, L. and R. Taylor (2002). Applying cluster analysis to define a typology of CFS in a medically evaluated, random community sample. *Psychology and Health,* 17(3):323-337.
13. Carruthers, B., M. van de Sande, K. De Meirleir, N. Klimas, G. Broderick, T. Mitchell, D. Staines, A. Powles, N. Speight, R. Vallings, L. Bateman, B. Baumgarten-Austrheim, D. Bell, N. Carlo-Stella, J. Chia, A. Darragh, D. Jo, D. Lewis, A. Light, S. Marshall-Gradisbik, I. Mena, J. Mikovits, K. Miwa, M. Murovska, M. Pall & S. Stevens (2017, p. 3). Myalgic encephalomyelitis: International Consensus Criteria. *Journal of Internal Medicine,* 282(4):353.
14. Brkic, S., S. Tomic, M. Ruzic & D. Maric (2011). Chronic Fatigue Syndrome. *Srpski Arhiv za Celokupno Lekarstvo,* 139(3-4):256.
15. Kraft, S. (2015). What is chronic fatigue syndrome? What causes chronic fatigue syndrome? *Medical News Today*, February 13, 2015. http://www.medicalnewstoday.com/articles/184802.
16. Jason, L. and J. Richman (2008). How science can stigmatize: The case of CFS. *Journal of CFS,* 14(4):85-103.

17. Institute of Medicine of the National Academies: Committee on the diagnostic criteria for ME/CFS (2015, p. 74). *Beyond ME/CFS: Redefining an illness.* Washington (DC): National Academies Press (US). February 2015.

18. Bazelmans, E., G. Bleijenberg, M.J. Voeten, J.W. Van Der Meer & H. Folgering (2005). Impact of maximal exercise test on symptoms and activity in CFS. *Journal of Psychosomatic Research* 59(4):201-208.

19. Arroll, M., E.A. Altree, J.M. O'Leary & C.P. Dancey (2014). The delayed fatigue effect in ME/CFS. *Fatigue: Biomedicine, Health & Behavior,* 2(2):57-63.

20. Davenport, T., S. Stevens, K. Baroni, M. Van Ness & C. Snell (2011). Diagnostic accuracy of symptoms characterizing CFS. *Disability & Rehabilitation,* 33(19-20):1768-1775.

21. Hossain J., P. Ahmad, L. Reinish, L. Kayumov, N. Hossain & C. Shapiro (2005). Subjective fatigue and subjective sleepiness: Two independent consequences of sleep disorders. *Journal of Sleep Research,* 14(3):245–253.

22. FDA (Food and Drug Administration) (2013). *The voice of the patient: CFS and ME.* Bethesda, MD: Center for Drug Evaluation and Research (CDER), FDA.

23. Peterson, P., S. Sirr, F. Grammith, C. Schenck, A. Pheley, S. Hu & C. Chao (2004). Effects of mild exercise on cytokines and cerebral blood flow in CFS patients. *Clinical and Diagnostic Laboratory Immunology,* 1(2):222-226.

24. vos-Vromans, D., I. Huijnen, A. Koke, H. Seelen, J. Knottnerus & R. Smeets (2013). Differences in physical functioning between relatively active and passive patients with Chronic Fatigue Syndrome. *Journal of Psychosomatic Research,* 75(3):249-254.

25. Meeus, M., I. Van Eupen, E. van Baarle, V. De Boeck, A. Luyck, D. Kos & J. Nijs (2011). Symptom fluctuations and daily physical activity in patients with CFS: A case-control study. *Physical medicine and rehabilitation,* 92(11):1820-1826.

26. Evering, R., R. Tonis & M. Vollenbroek-Hutton (2011). Deviations in daily physical activity patterns in patients with the CFS: A case control study. *Journal of Psychosomatic Research,* 71(3):129-135.

27. Jason, L. and M. Brown (2013). Sub-typing daily fatigue progression in CFS. *Journal of Mental Health,* 22(1):4-11.

28. Institute of Medicine of the National Academies: Committee on the diagnostic criteria for ME/CFS (2015, p. 86). *Beyond ME/CFS: Redefining an illness.* Washington (DC): National Academies Press (US). February 2015.

29. Cook, D., A. Light, K. Light, G. Broderick, M. Shields, R. Dougherty, J. Meyer, S. VanRiper, A. Stegner, L. Ellingson & S. Vernon (2017). Neural consequences of post-exertion malaise in Myalgic Encephalomyelitis/ Chronic Fatigue Syndrome. *Brain, Behavior, and Immunity,* 62:87-99. https://doi.org/10.1016/j.bbi.2017.02.009.

30. Nijs, J., J. Van Oosterwijck, M. Meeus, L. Lambrecht, K. Metzger, M. Fremont & L. Paul (2010). Unravelling the nature of postexertional malaise in ME/CFS: The role of elastase, complement C4a and inter-leukin-1beta. *Journal of Internal Medicine,* 267(4):418-435.

31. White, A., A. Light, R. Hughen, L. Bateman, T. Martins, H. Hill & K. Light (2010). Severity of symptoms flare after moderate exercise is linked to cytokine activity in CFS. *Psychophysiology,* 47(4):615-624.

32. Spotila, J. (2010). *Post-exertional malaise in CFS.* Charlotte, NC: CFIDS Association of America.

33. Van Ness, J., S. Stevens, L. Bateman, T. Stiles & C. Snell (2010). Post-exertional malaise in women with CFS. *Journal of Women's Health,* 19(2):239-244.

34. Meeus, M., L. Hermans, K. Ickmas, F. Struyf, D. Van Cauwenbergh, L. Bronckaerts, L. De Clerck, G. Moorken, G. Hans, S. Grosemans & J. Nijs (2014). Endogenous pain modulation in response to exercise in patients with rheumatoird arthritis, patients with CFS and comor-bid fibromyalgia, and healthy controls: A double-blind randomized controlled trial. *Pain Practice.* http://www:onlinelibrary.wiley. com/ doi/10.1111/papr.12181/pdf.

35. Ocon, A., Z. Messer, M. Medow & J. Stewart (2012). Increasing orthostatic stress impairs neurocognitive functioning in CFS with postural tachycardia syndrome. *Clinical Science,* 122(5):227-238.

36. Davenport, T., S. Stevens, K. Baroni, J. Van Ness & C. Snell (2011). Reliability and validity of Short Form 36 version 2 to measure health perceptions in a sub-group of individuals with fatigue. *Disability & Rehabilitation,* 33(25-26):2596-2604.

37. Kishi, A., F. Togo, D. Cook, M. Klapholz, Y. Yamamoto, D. Rapoport & B. Natelson (2013). The effects of exercise on dynamic sleep morphology in healthy controls and patients with CFS. *Psychological Reports,* 1(6): e00152.

38. Jones, D., K. Hollingsworth, R. Taylor, A. Blamire & J. Newton (2010). Abnormalities in ph handling by peripheral muscle and potential regulation by the autonomic nervous system in CFS. *Journal of Internal Medicine,* 267(4):394-401.

39. Meyer, J., A. Light, S. Shukla, D. Clevidence, S. Yale, A. Stegner & D. Cook (2013). Post-exertion malaise in CFS: Symptoms and gene expression. *Fatigue: Biomedicine, Health & Behavior,* 1(4):190-209.

40. Chou, K.L. (2013). Chronic fatigue and affective disorders in older adults: Evidence from the 2007 British National Psychiatric Morbidity Survey. *Journal of Affective Disorders,* 145(3):331-335.

41. Jason, L., N. Porter, J. Hunnell, A. Rademaker & J. Richman (2011). CFS prevalence and risk factors over time. *Journal of Health Psychology,* 16(3):120-135.

42. Zhang, L., J. Gough, D. Christmas, D. Mattey, S. Richards, J. Main, D. Enlander, D. Honeybourne, J. Ayres, D. Nutt & J. Kerr (2010). Microbial infections in eight genomic subtypes of CFS/ME. *Journal of Clinical Pathology,* 63(2):156-164.

43. Hawk, C., L. Jason & S. Torres-Harding (2006). Differential diagnosis of CFS and major depressive disorder. *International Journal of Behavioral Medicine,* 13(3):244-251.

44. Kerr, J., J. Gough, S. Richards, J. Main, D. Enlander, M. McCreary, A. Komaroff & J. Chia (2010). Antibody to parvovirus B19 nonstructural

protein is associated with chronic arthralgia in patients with CFS/ME. *Journal of General Virology,* 91(Pt. 4):893-897.

45. Chu, L., I. Valencia, D. Garvert & J. Montoya (2018). Deconstructing post-exertional malaise in myalgic encephalomyelitis/chronic fatigue syndrome: A patient-centered, cross-sectional survey. Plos One, Published: June 1, 2018, https://doi.org/10.1371/journal.pone.0197811.

46. Capuron, L., L. Welberg, C. Heim, D. Wagner, L. Solomon, D. Papanicolaou, R. Craddock, A. Miller & C. Reeves (2006). Cognitive dysfunction relates to subjective report of mental fatigue in patients with CFS. *Neuropsychopharmacology,* 31(8):1777-1784.

47. Light, A., L. Bateman, D. Jo, R. Hughen, T. Vanhaitsma, A. White & K. Light (2012). Gene expression alterations at baseline and following moderate exercise in patients with CFS and fibromyalgia syndrome. *Journal of Internal Medicine,* 271(1):64-81.

48. White, P., K. Goldsmith, A. Johnson, L. Potts, R. Walwyn, J.C. DeCesare, H. Baber, M. Burgess, L. Clark, D. Cox, J. Bavinton, B. Angus, G. Murphy, M. Murphy, H. O'Dowd, D. Wilks, P. McCrone, T. Chalder & M. Sharpe (2011). Comparison of adaptive pacing therapy, cognitive behavior therapy, graded exercise therapy, and specialist medical care for CFS: A randomized trial. *The Lancet,* 377(9768): 823-836.

49. Cockshell, S. and J. Mathias (2014). Cognitive functioning in people with CFS: A comparison between subjective and objective measures. *Neuropsychology,* 28(3):394-405.

50. Brenu, E., K. Ashton, M. van Driel, D. Staines, D. Peterson, G. Atkinson & S. Marshall-Gradisnik (2012). Cytotoxic lymphocyte microRNAs as prospective biomarkers for Chronic Fatigue Syndrome/Myalgic Encephalomyelitis. *Journal of Affective Disorders,* 141(2-3):261-9. doi: 10.1016/j.jad.2012.03.037.

51. Maes, M., F. Twisk, N. Kubera & N. Ringel (2012). Evidence for inflammation and activation of cell-mediated immunity in ME/CFS: Increased interleukin-1, tumor necrosis factor-a, PMN-elastase, lysozyme and neopterin. *Journal of Affective Disorders,* 136(3):933-939. doi: 10.1016/j.jad.2011.

52. Morris, G. and M. Maes (2012). Increased nuclear factor-kB and loss of p53 are key mechanisms in ME/CFS. *Medical Hypotheses,* 79(5):607-613.

53. Nijs, J., A. Nees, L. Paul, M. De Kooning, K. Ickmans, M. Meeus & J. Van Oosterwijck (2014). Alterered immune response to exercise in patients with CFS/ME: A systemic literature review. *Exercise Immunology Review,* 20:94-116.

54. Maes, M., F. Twisk, M. Kubera, K. Ringel, J-C. Leunis & M. Geffard (2012). Increased IgA responses to the LPS of commensal bacteria is associated with inflammation and activation of cell-mediated immunity in CFS. *Journal of Affective Disorders,* 136 (3):909-917.

55. Maes, M., F. Twisk & C. Johnson (2012). ME, CFS and Chronic Fatigue (CF) are distinguished accurately: Results of supervised learning techniques applies on clinical and inflammatory data. *Psychiatry Research*, 200(2-3):754-60. doi:10.1016/ j.psychres. 2012.03.031.

56. Taylor, R., L. Jason & C. Curie (2002). Prognosis of CFS in a community-based sample. *Psychosomatic Medicine,* 64(202):310-327.

57. Fossey, M., E. Libman, S. Bailes, M. Baltzan, R. Schondorf, R. Amsel & C. Fichten (2004). Sleep quality and psychological adjustment in CFS. *Journal of Behavioral Medicine,* 27(6):581-605.

58. Carruthers, B, A. Jain, K. De Meirleir, D. Peterson, N. Klimas, A. Lerner, A. Bested, P. Flor-Henry, P. Joshi, A. Powles & J. Sherkey (2003). Myalgic encephalomyelitis/chronic fatigue syndrome: clinical working case definition, diagnostic and treatment protocols. *Journal of chronic fatigue syndrome*, 11(1):107-115.

59. IACFS/ME (International Association for ME/CFS) (2012). *ME/CFS: A primer for clinical practitioners.* Chicago, IL: IACFS/ME.

60. LeBon, O., D. Neu, Y. Berquin, J-P. Lanquart, R. Hoffman, O. Mairesse & R. Armitage (2012). Ultra-slow delta power in CFS. *Psychiatry Research,* 200(2-3):742-747.

61. Armitage, R., C. Landis, R. Hoffmaan, M. Lentz, N. Watson, J. Goldberg & D. Buchwald (2009). Power spectral analysis of sleep EEG in twins discordant for CFS. *Journal of Psychosomatic Research,* 66(1):51-57.

62. Kishi, A., Z. Struzik, B. Natelson, F. Togo & Y. Yamamoto (2008). Dynamics of sleep stage transitions in healthy humans and patients with CFS. *American Journal of Physiology – Regulatory Integrative & Comparative Physiology,* 294(6): R1980-R1987.

63. Neu, D., O. Mairesse, G. Hoffman, A. Dris, L. Lambrecht, P. Linkowski, P. Verbanck & L. Olivier (2007). Sleep quality perception in the CFS: Correlations with sleep efficiency, affective symptoms and intensity of fatigue. *Neuropsychobiology,* 56(1):40-46.

64. Morriss, R., A. Wearden & L. Battersby (1997). The relation of sleep difficulties to fatigue, mood and disability in CFS. *Journal of Psychosomatic Research,* 42(6):597-605.

65. Nakamura. T., F. Togo, N. Cherniack, D. Rapoport & B. Natelson (2010). A subgroup of patients with CFS may have a disorder of arousal. *The Open Sleep Journal,* 3(6-11).

66. Burton, A., K. Rahman, Y. Kadota, A. Lloyd & M. Vollmer-Conna (2010). Reduced heart rate variability predicts poor sleep quality in a case-control study of CFS. *Experimental Brain Research,* 204(1):71-78.

67. Togo, F. and B. Natalson (2013). Heart rate variability during sleep and subsequent sleepiness in patients with CFS. *Autonomic Neuroscience: Basic and Clinical,* 1761(2):85-90.

68. Reeves, W., C. Heim, E. Maloney, L. Youngblood, E. Unger, M. Decker, J. Jones & D. Rye (2006). Sleep characteristics of persons with CFS and non-fatigued controls: Results from a population-based study. *BMC Neurology,* 6.

69. Creti, L., E. Libman, M. Baltzan, D. Rizzo, S. Bailes & C. Fichten (2010). Impaired sleep in CFS: How is it best measured? *Journal of Health Psychology,* 15(4):596-607.

70. Gotts, Z., V. Dreary, J. Newton, D. Van der Dussen, P. De Roy & J. Ellis (2013). Are there sleep-specific phenotypes in patients with CFS? A cross-sectional polysomnography analysis. *BMJ Open,* 3(6).

71. Cowan, D., G. Allardice, D. Macfarlane, D. Ramsay, H. Ambler, S. Banham, E. Livingston & C. Carlin (2014). Predicting sleep disordered breathing in outpatients with suspected OSA. *BMJ Open,* 4(4): e004519.

72. Mariman, A., L. Delesie, E. Tobback, I. Hanoulle, E. Sermijn, P. Vermeir, D. Pevernagie & D. Vogelaers (2013). Undiagnosed and comorbid disorders in patients with presumed CFS. *Journal of Psychosomatic Research,* 75(5):491-496.

73. Jason, L., M. Sunnquist, A. Brown, M. Evans, S. Vernon, J. Furst & V. Simonis (2013). Examining case definition criteria for CFS and ME. *Fatigue: Biomedicine, Health & Behavior,* 2(1).

74. Kushida, C., M. Littner, T. Morgenthaler, C. Alessi, D. Bailey, J. Coleman, Jr., L. Friedman, M. Hirshkowitz, S. Kapen, M. Kramer, T. Lee-Chiong, D. Loube, J. Owens, J. Pancer & M. Wise (2005). Practice parameters for the indications for polysomnography and related procedures: An update for 2005. *Sleep,* 28(4):499-521.

75. Jackson, M. and D. Bruck (2012). Sleep abnormalities in CFS/ME: A review. *Journal of Clinical Sleep Medicine,* 8(6):719-718.

76. Institute of Medicine of the National Academies: Committee on the diagnostic criteria for ME/CFS (2015, p. 96). *Beyond ME/CFS: Redefining an illness.* Washington (DC): National Academies Press (US). February 2015.

77. Quanneta, R. (2014). Obstructive sleep apnea syndrome manifested as a subset of CFS: A comorbidity or an exclusion criterion? *Rheumatology International,* 34(3):441-442.

78. Foral, P., J. Knezevich, N. Dewan & M. Malesker (2011). Medication-induced sleep disturbances. *The Consultant Pharmacist,* 26(6):414-425.

79. Kierlin, L. and M. Littner (2011). Parasomnias and antidepressant therapy: A review of the literature. *Front Psychiatry,* 2:71.

80. Cockshell, S. and J. Mathias (2010). Cognitive functioning in CFS: A meta-analysis. *Psychological Medicine,* 40(8):1253-1267.

81. Constant, E., S. Adam, B. Gillain, M. Lambert, E. Masquelier & S. Seron (2011). Cognitive deficits in patients with CFS compared to those with major depressive disorder and healthy controls. *Clinical Neurology Neurosurgery,* 113(4):295-302.

82. Van Den Eede, F., G. Moorkens, W. Hulstein, Y, Maas, D. Schrijvers, S. Stevens, P. Cosyns, S. Claes & B. Sabbe (2011). Psychomotor

function and response inhibition in CFS. *Psychiatry Research,* 186(2-3):367-372.

83. Schrijvers, D., F. Van Den Eede, Y. Maas, P. Cosyns, W. Hulstijn & B. Sabbe (2009). Psychomotor functioning in CFS and major depressive disorder: A comparative study. *Journal of Affective Disorders,* 115(1-2):46-53.

84. Cockshell, S. and J. Mathias (2014). Cognitive functioning in people with CFS: A comparison between subjective and objective measures. *Neuropsychology,* 28(3):394-405.

85. Cockshell, S., J. Mathias & S. Rao (2013). Cognitive deficits in CFS and their relationship to psychological status, symptomatology, and everyday functioning. *Neuropsychology,* 27(2):230-242.

86. Attree, E., C. Dancey & A. Pope (2009). An assessment of prospective memory retrieval in women with CFS using a virtual reality environment: An initial study. *Cyberpsychology and Behavior,* 12(4):379-385.

87. Hutchinson, C. and S. Badham (2013). Patterns of abnormal visual attention in ME. *Optometry and Vision Science,* 90(6):607-614.

88. Hou, R., R. Moss-Morris, A. Risdale, J. Lynch, P. Jeevaratnam, B. Bradley & K. Mogg (2014). Attention processes in CFS: Attentional bias for health-related threat and the role of attentional control. *Behavior Research and Therapy,* 52:9-16.

89. Nacul, L., E. Lacerda, D. Pheby, P. Campion, M. Drachler, J. Leite, F. Poland, A. Howe, S. Fayyaz & M. Molokhia (2011). The functional status and well-being of people with ME/CFS and their careers. *BMC Public Health,* 11(1):402.

90. Institute of Medicine of the National Academies: Committee on the diagnostic criteria for ME/CFS (2015, p. 107). *Beyond ME/CFS: Redefining an illness.* Washington (DC): National Academies Press (US). February 2015.

91. De Becker, P., N. McGregor & K. De Meirleir (2001). A definition-based analysis of symptoms in a large cohort of patients with CFS. *Journal of Internal Medicine,* 250(3):234-240.

92. Biswal, B., P. Kunwar & B. Natelson (2011). Cerebral blood flow is

reduced in CFS as assessed by arterial spin labelling. *Journal of the Neurological Sciences,* 301(1):9-11.

93. Majer, M., L. Welberg, L. Capuron, A. Miller, G. Pagnoni & W. Reeves (2008). Neuropsychological performance in persons with CFS: Results from a population-based study. *Psychosomatic Medicine,* 70(7):829-836.

94. Caseras, X., D. Mataix-Cols, V. Giampietro, K. Rimes, M. Brammer, F. Zelaya, T. Chalder & E. Godfrey (2006). Probing the working memory system in CFS: A functional magnetic resonance imaging study using the n-back task. *Psychosomatic Medicine,* 68(6):947-955.

95. Cook, D., P. O'Connor, G. Lange, and J. Steffener (2007). Functional neuroimaging correlates of mental fatigue induced by cognition among CFS patients and controls. *Neuroimage,* 36(1):108-122.

96. Lange, G., J. Steffener, D. Cook, B. Bly, C. Christodoulou, W. Liu, J. DeLuca & B. Natelson (2005). Objective evidence of cognitive complaints in CFS: A BOLD MRI study of verbal working memory. *Neuroimage,* 26(2):513-524.

97. De Lange, F., J. Kalkman, G. Bleijenberg, P. Hagoort, J. van der Meer & I. Toni (2015). Gray matter volume reduction in the CFS. *Neuroimage,* 26(3):777-781.

98. Barnden, L., B. Crouch, R. Kwiatek, R. Burnet, A. Mernone, S. Chryssidis, G. Scroop & P. del Fante (2011). A brain MRI study of CFS: Evidence of brainstem dysfunction and altered homeostasis. *NMR in Biomedicine,* 24(10):1302-1312.

99. Puri, B., P. Jakeman, M. Agour, K. Gunatilake, K. Fernando, A. Gurusinghe, I. Treasaden, A. Waldman & P. Gishen (2012). Regional grey and white matter volumetric changes in ME/CFS: A voxel-based morphometry 3 T MRI study. *British Journal of Radiology,* 85(1015):e270-e273.

100. Nakatomi, Y., K. Mizuno, A. Ishii, Y. Wada, M. Tanaka, S. Tazawa, K. Onoe, S. Fakuda, J. Kawabe, K. Takahashi, Y. Kataoka, S. Shiomi, K. Yamaguti, M. Inaba, H. Kuratsune & Y. Watanabe (2014). Neuroinflammation in patients with CFS/ME: An 11C-R-PK11195 PET study. *Journal of Nuclear Medicine,* 55(6):945-950.

101. Raj, S. (2013). Postural Orthostatic Tachycardia Syndrome (POTS). *Circulation,* 127(23):2336-2342.

102. CDC (Centers for disease control and prevention) (2012). Myalgic encephalomyelitis/chronic fatigue syndrome (ME/CFS). https://www.cdc.gov/me-cfs/index. (accessed 3/10/2015).

103. Gerrity, T., J. Bates, D. Bell, G. Chrousos, G. Furst, T. Hedrick, B. Hurwitz, R. Kyla, S. Levine, R. Moore & R. Schondorf (2002). CFS: What role does the autonomic nervous system play in the pathophysiology of this complex illness? *Neuroimmunomodulation,* 10(3):134-141.

104. Costigan, A., C. Elliott, C. McDonald & J. Newton (2010). Orthostatic symptoms predict functional capacity in CFS: Implications for management. *QJM: Monthly Journal of the Association of Physicians,* 103(8):589-595.

105. CDC (Centers for disease control and prevention) (2014). Recognition and management of CFS: A resource guide for health care professionals. http://www.cdc.gov/cfs/toolkit. (accessed 3/10/2015).

106. Low, P., P. Sandroni, M. Joyner & W. Shen (2009). Postural tachycardia syndrome. *Journal of Cardiovascular Electrophysiology,* 20(3).

107. FDA (Food and Drug Administration) (2013, p. 7). *The voice of the patient: CFS and ME.* Bethesda, MD: Center for Drug Evaluation and Research (CDER), FDA.

108. Hollingsworth, K., D. Jones, R. Taylor, A. Blamire & J. Newton (2010). Impaired cardiovascular response to standing in CFS. *European Journal of Clinical Investigation,* 40(7):608-615.

109. Miwa, K. (2014). Cardiac dysfunction and orthostatic intolerance in patients with ME and a small left ventricle. *Heart Vessels,* April 16, 2014.

110. Bou-Holaigah, I., P. Rowe, J. Kan & H. Calkins (1995). The relationship between neutrally mediated hypotension and the CFS. *Journal of the American Medical Association,* 274(12):961-967.

111. Newton, J., O. Konkwo, K. Sutcliffe, A. Seth, J. Shin and D. Jones (2007). Symptoms of autonomic dysfunction in chronic fatigue syndrome. *JM: Monthly Journal of the Association of Physicians,* 100(8):519-526.

112. Hurwitz, B., V. Coryell, M. Parker, P. Martin, A. Laperriere, N. Klimas, G. Sfakianakis & M. Bilsker (2010). CFS: Illness severity, sedentary lifestyle, blood volume and evidence of diminished cardiac function. *Clinical Science,* 118(2):125-135.

113. Streeten, D. and D. Bell (1998). Circulating blood volume in CFS. *Journal of CFS,* 4(1):3-11.

114. Okamoto, L., S. Raj, A. Peltier, A. Gamboa, C. Shibao, A. Diedrich, B. Black, D. Robertson & I. Biaggioni (2012). Neurohumoral and haemodynamic profile in postural tachycardia and CFS. *Clinical Science,* 122(4):183-192.

115. Newton, D., G. Kennedy, K. Chan, C. Lang, J. Belch & F. Khan (2012). Cardiovascular risk: Large and small artery endothelial dysfunction in chronic fatigue syndrome. *International Journal of Cardiology*, 154(3):335-6. doi: 10.1016/j.ijcard.2011.10.030.

Chapter 5

1. Cella, M., M. Sharpe & T. Chalder (2011). Measuring disability in patients with CFS: Reliability and validity of the work and social adjustment scale. *Journal of Psychosomatic Research*, 71(3):124-128.

2. Institute of Medicine of the National Academies: Committee on the diagnostic criteria for ME/CFS (2015). *Beyond ME/CFS: Redefining an illness*. Washington (DC): National Academies Press (US). February 2015.

3. University of Maryland Medical System (2013, p. 10). *Chronic Fatigue Syndrome: An in-depth report on the causes, diagnosis and treatment of CFS.* http://umm.edu/health/medical/reports/articles/chronic-fatigue-syndrome/. (accessed 3-11-2015).

4. NIH (National Institute of Health) (2011). *State of the knowledge workshop. ME/CFS research: Workshop report.* Bethseda, MD: Office of Research on Women's Health, NIH, US Department of Health and Human Services.

5. Chou, K.L. (2013). Chronic fatigue and affective disorders in older adults: Evidence from the 2007 British National Psychiatric Morbidity Survey. *Journal of Affective Disorders*, 145(3):331-335.

6. Carruthers, B., M. van de Sande, K. De Meirleir, N. Klimas, G. Broderick, T. Mitchell, D. Staines, A. Powles, N. Speight, R. Vallings, L. Bateman, B. Baumgarten-Austrheim, D. Bell, N. Carlo-Stella, J. Chia, A. Darragh, D. Jo, D. Lewis, A. Light, S. Marshall-Gradisbik, I. Mena, J. Mikovits, K. Miwa, M. Murovska, M. Pall & S. Stevens (2017). Myalgic encephalomyelitis: International Consensus Criteria. *Journal of Internal Medicine,* 282(4):353.

7. vos-Vromans, D., I. Huijnen, A. Koke, H. Seelen, J. Knottnerus & R. Smeets (2013). Differences in physical functioning between relatively active and passive patients with Chronic Fatigue Syndrome. *Journal of Psychosomatic Research,* 75(3):249-254.

8. Jason, L. and J. Richman (2008). How science can stigmatize: The case of CFS. *Journal of CFS,* 14(4):85-103.

9. Kraft, S. (2015). What is chronic fatigue syndrome? What causes chronic fatigue syndrome? *Medical News Today,* February 13, 2015. http://www.medicalnewstoday.com/articles/184802.

10. Evering, R., R. Tonis & M. Vollenbroek-Hutton (2011). Deviations in daily physical activity patterns in patients with the chronic fatigue syndrome: A case control study. *Journal of Psychosomatic Research,* 71(3):129-135.

11. IDAC (Invisible Disabilities Association of Canada) (2012). Chronic Fatigue Syndrome/Myalgic Encephalomyelitis: Definition, diagnosis, symptoms and treatment. http://www.disabilityliving.ca/disability-canada-invisible-disabilities-association-resources/.

12. New York Times Health (2009). Chronic Fatigue: In-depth report. The New York Times Health. http://www.nytimes.com/health/guides/disease/chronic-fatigue-syndrome. (accessed 3/10/15).

13. Wiborg, J., S. van der Werf, J. Prins & G. Bleijenberg (2010). Being homebound with CFS: A multidimensional comparison with outpatients. *Psychiatry Research,* 177(1-2):246-249.

14. Taylor, R. and G. Kielhofner (2005). Work related impairment and employment-focused rehabilitation options for individuals with CFS: A review. *Journal of Mental Health,* 14(3):253-267.

15. Chu, L., I. Valencia, D. Garvert & J. Montoya (2019). Onset patterns

and course of ME/CFS. *Frontiers in Pediatrics*, February 5, 2019, https://doi.org/10.3389/fped.2019.00012.

16. Reynolds, K., S. Vernon, E. Bouchery & W. Reeves (2004). The economic impact of CFS. *Cost Effectiveness and Resource Allocation,* 2(4).

17. Jason, L., M. Benton, L. Valentine, A. Johnson & S. Torres-Harding (2008). The economic impact of ME/CFS: Individual and societal costs. *Dynamic Medicine*, 7(1).

18. Lin, J., S. Resch, D. Brimmer, A. Johnson, S. Kennedy, N. Burstein & C. Simon (2011). The economic impact of CFS in Georgia: Direct and indirect costs. *Cost effectiveness and Resource Allocation,* 9(1).

19. Valdez, A., E. Hancock, S. Adebayo, D. Kiernicki, D. Proskauer, J. Attewell, L. Bateman, A. DeMaria, C. Lapp, P. Rowe & C. Proskauer (2019). Estimating prevalence, demographics, and costs of ME/CFS using large scale medical claims data and machine learning. *Frontiers in Pediatrics*, 2018, 6:412. Published online January 8, 2019. doi: 10.3389/fped.2018.00412.

20. Mariman, A., L. Delesie, E. Tobback, I. Hanoulle, E. Sermijn, P. Vermeir, D. Pevernagie & D. Vogelaers (2013). Undiagnosed and comorbid disorders in patients with presumed CFS. *Journal of Psychosomatic Research,* 75(5):491-496.

21. Park, J. and Gilmour H. (2017). *MUPS among adults in Canada: Comorbidity, health care use and employment.* Statistics Canada, catalogue no. 82-003-X, ISSN 1209-1367, Health Reports, Vol. 28, no. 3, pp. 3-8, March 2017.

22. Deary, V. and T. Chalder (2010). Personality and perfectionism in CFS: A closer look. *Psychology and Health,* 25(4):465-475.

23. Chang, C., J. Warren & E. Engels (2012). Chronic fatigue syndrome and subsequent risk of cancer among elderly U.S. adults. *Cancer*, 118(23):5929-5936. Doi: 10.1002/cncr.27612.

24. Newton, D., G. Kennedy, K. Chan, C. Lang, J. Belch & F. Khan (2012). Cardiovascular risk: Large and small artery endothelial dysfunction in chronic fatigue syndrome. *International Journal of Cardiology*, 154(3):335-6. doi: 10.1016/j.ijcard.2011.10.030.

25. Witham, M., G. Kennedy, J. Belch & F. Khan (2014). Association between vitamin D status and markers of vascular health in patients with CFS/ME. *International Journal of Cardiology,* 174(1):139-140.

26. Carruthers, B. and M. van de Sande (2005). *ME/CFS: A clinical case definition and guidelines for medical practitioners: An overview of the Canadian Consensus Document.* Haworth Medical Press Inc., Canada.

27. Jason, L., K. Corradi, S. Gress, S. Williams & S. Torres-Harding (2006). Causes of death among patients with chronic fatigue syndrome. *Health care for women international,* 27(7):615–626. doi:10.1080/07399330600803766.

28. Jason, L., M. Brown, M. Evans, V. Anderson, A. Lerch, A. Brown, J. Hunnell & N. Porter (2011). Measuring substantial reductions in functioning in patients with CFS. *Disability and Rehabilitation,* 33(7):589-598.

29. Brooks, S., J. Daglish & A. Wearden (2013). Attributions, distress and behavioral responses in the significant others of people with CFS. *Journal of Health Psychology,* 18(10):1288-1295.

30. Band, R., C. Barrowclough, A. Wearden & A. Kazak (2014). The impact of significant other expressed emotion on patient outcomes in CFS. *Health Psychology,* 33(9):1092-1101.

31. Anderson, V., M. Maes & M. Berk (2012). Biological underpinnings of the commonalities of depression, somatization and CFS. *Medical Hypotheses,* 78(6):752-756.

32. Anderson, V., L. Jason, L. Hlavaty, N. Porter & J. Cudia (2012). A review and meta-synthesis of qualitative studies in ME/CFS, *Patient Education and Counseling,* 86(2):147-155.

33. Arroll, M. and A. Howard (2013). The letting go, the building up, and the gradual process of rebuilding: Identity change and post-traumatic growth in ME/CFS. *Psychology and Health,* 28(3):302-318.

34. Larun, L. and K. Malterud (2007). Identity and coping experiences in CFS: A synthesis of qualitative studies. *Patient Education and Counselling,* 69(1-3):20-28.

35. Nacul, L., E. Lacerda, D. Pheby, P. Campion, M. Drachler, J. Leite, F. Poland, A. Howe, S. Fayyaz & M. Molokhia (2011). The functional

status and well-being of people with ME/CFS and their careers. *BMC Public Health,* 11(1):402.

36. Tremlow, S., S. Bradshaw, Jr., L. Coyne & B. Lerma (1997). Patterns of utilization of medical care and perceptions of the relationship between doctor and patient with chronic illness including CFS. *Psychological Reports,* 80(2):643-658.

37. Twisk, F. (2017). Dangerous exercise: The detrimental effects of exertion and orthostatic stress in myalgic encephalomyelitis and chronic fatigue syndrome. *Physical Medicine and Rehabilitative Research:*February, 2017. http://dx/doi.org/10.15761/ PMRR.1000134.

38. Jason, L., E. Paavola, N. Porter & M. Morello (2010). Frequency and content analysis of CFS in medical textbooks. *Australian Journal of Primary Health,* 16(2):174-178.

39. Peterson, T., T.W. Peterson, S. Emerson, E. Regalbuto, M. Evans & L. Jason (2013). Coverage of CFS within U.S. medical schools. *Universal Journal of Public Health,* 1(4):177-179.

40. Jason, L., M. Evans, N. Porter, M. Brown, A. Brown, J. Hannell, V. Anderson, A. Lerch, K. De Meirleir & F. Friedberg (2010). The development of the revised Canadian ME/CFS case definition. *American Journal of Biochemistry and Biotechnology,* 6:120-135.

41. Dimmock, M., M. Mirin & L. Jason (2016). Estimating the disease burden of ME/CFS in the United States and its relation to research funding. *Journal of Medical Therapy,* 1: DOI: 10.15761/JMT.1000102.

42. McGrath, S. (2018b, p. 1). There is a yawning gap in ME/CFS research funding: Take action. http://www:mecfsresearch.me/2018/05/08/thereis-a-yawning-gap-in-me-cfs-research-funding-take-action.

43. CDC (Centers for disease control and prevention) (2012). Myalgic encephalomyelitis/chronic fatigue syndrome (ME/CFS). https://www.cdc.gov/me-cfs/index. (accessed 3/10/2015).

44. IACFS/ME (International Association for ME/CFS) (2012). *ME/CFS: A primer for clinical practitioners.* Chicago, IL: IACFS/ME.

45. Knoop, H. and J. Wiborg (2015). What makes a difference in CFS? *The Lancet Psychiatry,* 2(2):113-114.

46. Brown, M., D. Bell, L. Jason, C. Christos & D. Bell (2012).

Understanding long-term outcomes of CFS. *Journal of Clinical Psychology,* 68(9):1028(8).

47. Collin, S. and E. Crawley (2017). Specialist treatment of CFS/ME: A cohort study among adult patients in England. *BMC Health Services Research,* 17(1):488.

48. Andersen, M., H. Permin & F. Albrecht, F. (2004). Illness and disability in Danish Chronic Fatigue Syndrome patients at diagnosis and 5-year follow-up. *Journal of Psychosomatic Research,* 56(2):217–229. doi:10.1016/S0022-3999(03)00065-5.

49. Edwards, J., S. McGrath, A. Baldwin, M. Livingstone & A. Kewley (2016, p. 69). The biological challenges of ME/CFS: A solvable problem. *Fatigue,* 4(2): 63-69. doi:10.1080/21641846.2016.1160598.

Chapter 6

1. IACFS/ME (International Association for ME/CFS) (2012). *ME/CFS: A primer for clinical practitioners.* Chicago, IL: IACFS/ME.

2. Mayo Clinic (2014). Diseases and conditions: Chronic fatigue syndrome. http://www.mayoclinic.org/diseases-conditions/chronicfatiguesyndrome/ basics. (accessed April 4, 2015).

3. The Lancet (2015). What's in a name? Systemic exertion intolerance disease. *The Lancet,* February, 385(9969):663.

4. University of Maryland Medical System (2013). *Chronic Fatigue Syndrome: An in-depth report on the causes, diagnosis and treatment of CFS.* http://umm.edu/health/medical/reports/articles/chrnic-fatigue-syndrome/. (Accessed 3-10-2015).

5. Perry, S. and A. Santhouse (2012). Chronic Fatigue Syndrome. *Medicine,* 40(12):647-649.

6. Kraft, S. (2015). What is chronic fatigue syndrome? What causes chronic fatigue syndrome? *Medical News Today,* February 13, 2015. http://www.medicalnewstoday.com/articles/184802.

7. CDC (Centers for disease control and prevention) (2012). Myalgic encephalomyelitis/chronic fatigue syndrome (ME/CFS). https://www.cdc.gov/me-cfs/index. (accessed 3/10/2015).

8. Knoop, H., J. Prins, R. Moss-Morris & G. Bleijenberg (2010).

The central role of cognitive processes in the perpetuation of CFS. *Journal of Psychosomatic Research,* 68(5):489-494.

9. Wiborg, J., H. Knoop, L. Frank & G. Bleijenberg (2012). Towards an evidence-based treatment model for cognitive behavioral interventions focusing on CFS. *Journal of Psychosomatic Research,* 72(5):399-404.

10. Brooks, S., K. Rimes & T. Chalder (2011). The role of acceptance in CFS. *Journal of Psychosomatic Research,* 71(6):411-415.

11. Brown, M., A. Brown & L. Jason (2010). Illness duration and coping style in CFS. *Psychological Reports,* 106(2):383(11).

12. Poppe, C., M. Petrovic, D. Vogelaers & G. Crombez (2013). Cognitive behavior therapy in patients with CFS: The role of illness acceptance and neuroticism. *Journal of Psyhosomatic Research,* 74(5):367-372.

13. Wiborg, J., H. Knoop, M. Stulemeijer, J. Prins & G. Bleijenberg (2010). How does cognitive behavioral therapy reduce fatigue in patients with CFS? The role of physical activity. *Psychological Medicine,* 40(8):1281-1287.

14. Chalder, T., K. Goldsmith, P. White, M. Sharpe & A. Pickles (2015). Rehabilitative therapies for CFS: A secondary mediation analysis of the PACE trial. *The Lancet Psychiatry,* 2(2):141-152.

15. Wearden, A., R. Emsley & A. Nezu (2013). Mediators of the effects on fatigue of pragmatic rehabilitation for CFS. *Journal of Consulting and Clinical Psychology,* 81(5):831-838.

16. Lopez, C., M. Antoni, F. Penedo, D. Weiss, S. Cruess, M-C. Segotas, L. Helder, S. Siegel, N. Klimas & M-A. Fletcher (2011). A pilot study of cognitive behavioral stress management effects on stress, quality of life, and symptoms in persons with CFS. *Journal of Psychosomatic Research,* 70(4):328-334.

17. Hall, D., E. Lattie, M. Antoni, M-A. Fletcher, S. Czaja, D. Perdomo & N. Klimas (2014). Stress management skills, cortisol awakening response and post exertional malaise in CFS. *Psychoneuroendocrinology,* 49:26-31.

18. Powell, D., C. Liossi, R. Moss-Morris & W. Schlotz (2013). Unstimulated cortisol secretory activity in everyday life and its

relationship with fatigue and CFS: A systemic review and subset meta-analysis. *Psychoneuroendocrinology,* 38:2405-2422.

19. Roberts, A., M. Charler, A. Papadopoulos, S. Wessely, T. Chalder & A. Cleare (2010). Does hypocortisolism predict a poor response to cognitive behavioraial therapy in CFS? *Psychological Medicine,* 40(3):515-522.

20. Carruthers, B. and M. van de Sande (2005). *ME/CFS: A clinical case definition and guidelines for medical practitioners: An overview of the Canadian Consensus Document.* Haworth Medical Press Inc., Canada.

21. Carruthers, B. and M. van de Sande (2005, p. 11). *ME/CFS: A clinical case definition and guidelines for medical practitioners: An overview of the Canadian Consensus Document.* Haworth Medical Press Inc., Canada.

22. Schreurs, K., M. Veehof, L. Passage & M. Vollenbroek-Hutton (2011). Cognitive behavioral treatment for CFS in a rehabilitation setting: Effectiveness and predictors of outcome. *Behavior Research and Therapy,* 49(12):908-913.

23. Flo, E. and T. Chalder (2014). Prevalence and predictors of recovery from CFS in a routine clinical practice. *Behavior Research and Therapy,* 63:1-8.

24. Knoop, H. and J. Wiborg (2015). What makes a difference in CFS? *The Lancet Psychiatry,* 2(2):113-114.

25. Kindlon, T. (2017). Treatment and management of CFS/ME: All roads lead to Rome. *Journal of Health Psychology*, 2(9):1146-1154.

26. Kindlon, T. (2011). The PACE trial in CFS. *The Lancet,* 377(9780):1833.

27. Whilshire, C., T. Kindlon, A. Matthees & S. McGrath (2017). Can patients with chronic fatigue syndrome really recover after graded exercise or cognitive behavioural therapy? A critical commentary and preliminary re-analysis of the PACE trial. *Fatigue: Biomedicine, Health & Behavior,* 5(1):43-56. Published online: 14-12-2016.

28. MEAssociation(2015). Pacetrialtreatments. https://www.meassociation. org.uk/2015/10/press-release-me-association-pace-trial-treatments).

29. ME Association (2015). Challenging the PACE trial follow-up report. *The Lancet, Psychiatry*, October 28, 2015.

30. Twisk, F. (2016). PACE: CBT and GET are not rehabilitative therapies. *The Lancet Psychiatry,* 3(2):PE6. http://doi.org/10.1016/S2215-0366(15)00554-4.

31. Dougall, D., A. Johnson, K. Goldsmith, M. Sharpe, B. Angus, T. Chalder & P. White (2014). Adverse events and deterioration reported by participants in the PACE trial of therapies for CFS. *Journal of Psychosomatic Research,* 77(1):20-26.

32. Brown, M., D. Bell, L. Jason, C. Christos & D. Bell (2012). Understanding long-term outcomes of CFS. *Journal of Clinical Psychology,* 68(9):1028(8).

33. CDC (Centers for disease control and prevention) (2018). Clinical care of patients with ME/CFS. https://www.cdc.gov/me-cfs/healthcare-providers/clinical-care-patients-mecfs. (accessed 12-07-2018).

34. Seltzer, J. (2018). Information for healthcare providers. https://me-pedia.org/wiki/info-for-healthcare-providers (July 29, 2018).

35. Reymeyer, J. and D. Tuller (2017). *Why did it take the CDC so long to reverse course on debunked treatments for chronic fatigue syndrome?* September 25, 2017. https://www.statnews.com/2017/09/25/chronic-fatigue-syndrome-CDC/.

36. Dimmock, M. (2018). Clinical guidance for ME: Evidence based guidance gone awry. www.meaction.net/2018/02/05/the-failure-of-clinical-guidance-for-people-with/me.

37. ME Association (2017). Guide to ME/CFS symptom/management: Part one. http://meassociation.org.uk/2017/07/me-association-guide-to-me-cfs-symptom-management-part-one-06-july-2017.

38. New York Times Health (2009). *Chronic Fatigue: In-depth report.* The New York Times Health. http://www.nytimes.com/health/guides/disease/chronic-fatigue-syndrome. (accessed 3/10/15).

39. CDC (Centers for disease control and prevention) (2019). What is ME/CFS. https://www.cdc.gov/me-cfs/about/index.html (accessed 19-05-2019).

40. Foral, P., J. Knezevich, N. Dewan & M. Malesker (2011). Medication-induced sleep disturbances. *The Consultant Pharmacist,* 26(6): 414-425.

41. Kierlin, L. and M. Littner (2011). Parasomnias and antidepressant therapy: A review of the literature. *Front Psychiatry,* 2:71.

42. Fluge, O., O. Bruland, K. Risa, A. Storstein, E. Kristoffersen, D. Sapkota, H. Naess, O. Dahl, H. Nyland, O. Mella & M. Reindl (2011). Benefit from B-Lymphoyte Depletion Using the Anti-CD Antibody Rituximab in CFS: A Double-Blind and Placebo-Controlled Study (B-Cell Depletion in CFS). *PloS One,* 6(10):e26358.

43. Bou-Holaigah, I., P. Rowe, J. Kan & H. Calkins (1995). The relationship between neutrally mediated hypotension and the chronic fatigue syndrome. *Journal of the American Medical Association,* 274(12):961-967.

44. Chu, L., I. Valencia, D. Garvert & J. Montoya (2019). Onset patterns and course of ME/CFS. *Frontiers in Pediatrics,* February 5, 2019, https://doi.org/10.3389/fped.2019.00012.

45. CDC (Centers for disease control and prevention) (2014). Recognition and management of CFS: A resource guide for health care professionals. http://www.cdc.gov/cfs/toolkit. (accessed 3/10/2015).

46. IDAC (Invisible Disabilities Association of Canada) (2012). Chronic Fatigue Syndrome/Myalgic Encephalomyelitis: Definition, diagnosis, symptoms and treatment. http://www.disabilityliving.ca/disability-canada-invisible-disabilities-association-resources/.

47. Wang, Y.Y., X. Li, J.P. Liu, H. Luo, L. Ma & T. Altraek (2014). Traditional Chinese medicine for CFS: A systematic review of randomized clinical trials. *Complementary Therapies in Medicine,* 22(4):826-833.

Chapter 7

1. Institute of Medicine of the National Academies: Committee on the diagnostic criteria for ME/CFS (2015, p. 5). *Beyond ME/CFS: Redefining an illness.* Washington (DC): National Academies Press (US). February 2015.

2. ME Action (2019, p. 1). What is ME/CFS. https://www.meaction.net/about/what-is-me/. (accessed 2019-05-19).

3. McGrath, S. (2018b, p. 1). There is a yawning gap in ME/CFS research funding: Take action. http://www:mecfsresearch.me/ 2018/05/08/thereis-a-yawning-gap-in-me-cfs-research-funding-take-action.

Appendix A:
ME/CFS Case Definitions/Criteria

Over the years, a number of clinical case definitions/criteria have been developed to facilitate medical professionals in diagnosing patients and researchers in undertaking studies. The more commonly used definitions, for both clinical and research purposes, are the Fakuda and Canadian Census Criteria (CCC). The British National Institute for Health and Clinical Excellence (NICE) and the International Consensus Criteria are also the more commonly used of the definitions [1, 2]. Each of these definitions/criteria will be addressed sequentially in the following text.

1. **Fakuda/U.S. Centers for Disease Control and Prevention (CDC) Case Definition:**

The Fakuda/CDC definition is the most widely used in patient clinical evaluations and in research studies [3]. According to this definition, fatigue is defined as a "self-reported persistent or relapsing fatigue lasting 6 or more consecutive months". To be diagnosed with ME/CFS, a patient would need to meet this definition of fatigue and undergo a clinical evaluation as follows:

a) *Fakuda guidelines for the evaluation and study of ME/CFS:*
A thorough medical history, physical examination, mental status examination and laboratory tests must be conducted to identify underlying or contributing conditions that require treatment. Diagnosis or classification cannot be made without such an evaluation. Clinically evaluated, unexplained chronic fatigue cases can be classified as chronic fatigue syndrome, if the patient meets both the following criteria:

i. clinically evaluated, unexplained persistent or relapsing chronic fatigue that is of a new or definite onset (i.e., not life-long), is not the result of ongoing exertion, is not substantially alleviated by rest, and results in substantial reductions in previous levels of occupational, educational, social, or personal activities, and

ii. the concurrent occurrence of four or more of the following symptoms:
- substantial impairment in short-term memory or concentration,
- sore throat,
- tender lymph nodes,
- muscle pain,
- multi-joint pain without swelling or redness,
- headaches of a new type, pattern, or severity,
- unrefreshing sleep, and
- post-exertional malaise lasting more than 24 hours.

These symptoms must have persisted or recurred during 6 or more consecutive months of illness and must not have predated the fatigue.

b) *conditions that exclude a diagnosis of ME/CFS:*
i. any active medical condition that may explain the presence of chronic fatigue, such as untreated hypothyroidism, sleep apnea and narcolepsy, and iatrogenic conditions such as side effects of medication,

ii. some diagnosable illnesses may relapse or may not have completely resolved during treatment. If the persistence of such a condition could explain the presence of chronic fatigue, and if it cannot be clearly established that the original condition has completely resolved with treatment, then such patients should not be classified as having CFS. Examples of illnesses that can present such a picture include some types of malignancies and chronic cases of hepatitis B or C virus infection,

iii. any past or current diagnosis of a major depressive disorder with psychotic or melancholic features:
- bipolar affective disorders,
- schizophrenia of any subtype,
- delusional disorders of any subtype,
- dementias of any subtype,
- anorexia nervosa, or
- bulimia nervosa,

iv. alcohol or other substance abuse, occurring within 2 years of the onset of chronic fatigue and any time afterwards, and

v. severe obesity as defined by a body mass index [body mass index = weight in kilograms ÷ (height in meters) equal to or greater than 45. [Note: body mass index values vary considerably among different age groups and populations. No "normal" or "average" range of values can be suggested in a fashion that is meaningful. The range of 45 or greater was selected because it clearly falls within the range of severe obesity].

Any unexplained abnormality detected on examination or other testing that strongly suggests an exclusionary condition must be resolved before attempting further classification.

c) *conditions that do not exclude a diagnosis of ME/CFS:*

i. any condition defined primarily by symptoms that cannot be confirmed by diagnostic laboratory tests, including fibromyalgia, anxiety disorders, somatoform disorders, nonpsychotic or melancholic depression, neurasthenia and multiple chemical sensitivity disorder,

ii. any condition under specific treatment, sufficient to alleviate all symptoms related to that condition and for which the adequacy of treatment has been documented. Such conditions include hypothyroidism for which the adequacy of replacement hormone has been verified by normal thyroid-stimulating hormone levels, or asthma in which the adequacy of treatment has been determined by pulmonary function and other testing,

iii. any condition, such as Lyme disease or syphilis, that was treated with definitive therapy before development of chronic symptoms, and

iv. any isolated and unexplained physical examination finding, or laboratory or imaging test abnormality that is insufficient to strongly suggest the existence of an exclusionary condition. Such conditions include an elevated antinuclear antibody titer that is inadequate, without additional laboratory or clinical evidence, to strongly support a diagnosis of a discrete connective tissue disorder.

d) *a note on the use of laboratory tests in the diagnosis of ME/CFS:*
A minimum battery of laboratory screening tests should be performed. Routinely performing other screening tests for all patients has no known value. However, further tests may be indicated on an individual basis to confirm or exclude another diagnosis, such as multiple sclerosis. In these cases, additional tests should be done according to accepted clinical standards. The use of tests to diagnose ME/CFS (as opposed to excluding other diagnostic possibilities) should be done only in the setting of protocol-based research. The fact that such tests are investigational and do not aid in diagnosis or management should be explained to the patient.

In clinical practice, no tests can be recommended for the specific purpose of diagnosing chronic fatigue syndrome. Tests should be directed toward confirming or excluding other possible clinical conditions. Examples of specific tests that do not confirm or exclude the diagnosis of chronic fatigue syndrome include serologic tests for Epstein-Barr virus, enteroviruses, retroviruses, human herpesvirus 6, and Candida albicans; tests of immunologic function, including cell population and function studies; and imaging studies, including magnetic resonance imaging scans and radionuclide scans (such as single-photon emission computed tomography and positron emission tomography) [4, 5].

2. Canadian Consensus Criteria (CCC) Case Definition:

The CCC definition is intended to improve diagnostic reliability and facilitate research studies as well. According to the CCC definition, a ME/CFS diagnosis would require:

1. the presence of fatigue, including a substantial reduction in activity level,
2. post exertional malaise (PEM) and/or post-exertional fatigue,
3. sleep dysfunction such as unrefreshing sleep or a disturbance of sleep quantity,
4. pain (or discomfort) that is often widespread and migratory in nature, and
5. symptoms from the following symptom categories for a period of 6 months or longer but not lifelong (i.e., the disease had an identifiable starting time):
   a) neurologic/cognitive manifestation symptom category (2 or more manifestations), and
   b) autonomic, neuroendocrine, or immune manifestation symptom category (at least 1 or more symptoms from 2 of these 3 categories).

   a) The neurological/cognitive manifestations include:
   confusion, impairment of concentration and short-term memory consolidation; disorientation, difficulty with information processing, categorizing and word retrieval; and perceptual and sensory disturbances (e.g., spatial instability and disorientation, and inability to focus vision). Ataxia, muscle weakness and fasciculations would also be common. There may also be a phenomenon of overload: cognitive, sensory (e.g., photophobia) and hypersensitivity to noise and/or emotional overload, which may lead to crash periods and/or anxiety.

   b) The autonomic, neuroendocrine, or immune manifestations include:

i. autonomic manifestations: orthostatic intolerance, neu-
    rally -mediated hypotension (NMH), postural orthostatic
    tachycardia syndrome (POTS), delayed postural hypoten-
    sion, light-headedness, extreme pallor, nausea and irritable
    bowel syndrome, urinary frequency and bladder dysfunc-
    tion, palpitations with or without cardiac arrhythmias, and
    exertional dyspnea,

ii. neuroendocrine manifestations: loss of thermostatic sta-
    bility, subnormal body temperature and marked diurnal
    fluctuation, sweating episodes, recurrent feelings of fever-
    ishness and cold extremities, intolerance of extremes of
    heat and cold, marked weight change, anorexia or abnor-
    mal appetite, loss of adaptability and worsening of symp-
    toms with stress, and

iii. immune manifestations: tender lymph nodes, recur-
     rent sore throat, recurrent flu-like symptoms, general
     malaise, new sensitivities to food, medications and/or
     chemicals [6].

3. United Kingdom's National Institute for Health and Clinical Excellence (NICE) Clinical Guidelines for ME/CFS:

The NICE definition is intended to facilitate the diagnosis and management
of ME/CFS. Healthcare professionals should consider the possibility of
ME/CFS if a person has:

- fatigue with all the following features:
  - new or had a specific onset (that is, it is not lifelong),
  - persistent and/or recurrent,
  - unexplained by other conditions,
  - has resulted in a substantial reduction in activity level, and
  - characterized by post-exertional malaise and/or fatigue
    (typically delayed, for example by at least 24 hours, with slow
    recovery over several days), and

- one or more of the following symptoms:
  - difficulty with sleeping, such as insomnia, hypersomnia, unrefreshing sleep, a disturbed sleep–wake cycle,
  - muscle and/or joint pain that is multi-site and without evidence of inflammation,
  - headaches,
  - painful lymph nodes without pathological enlargement,
  - sore throat,
  - cognitive dysfunction, such as difficulty thinking, inability to concentrate, impairment of short-term memory, and difficulties with word-finding, planning/organizing thoughts and information processing,
  - physical or mental exertion makes symptoms worse,
  - general malaise or 'flu-like' symptoms,
  - dizziness and/or nausea, and
  - palpitations in the absence of identified cardiac pathology.

Healthcare professionals should be aware that the symptoms of ME/CFS fluctuate in severity and may change in nature over time.

Signs and symptoms that can be caused by other serious conditions ('red flags') should not be attributed to ME/CFS without consideration of alternative diagnoses or comorbidities. In particular, the following features should be investigated:

- localizing/focal neurological signs,
- signs and symptoms of inflammatory arthritis or connective tissue disease,
- signs and symptoms of cardiorespiratory disease,
- significant weight loss,
- sleep apnea, and
- clinically significant lymphadenopathy.

A diagnosis should be made after other possible diagnoses have been excluded and the symptoms have persisted for:

163

- 4 months in an adult, and
- 3 months in a child or young person; the diagnosis should be made or confirmed by a pediatrician.

The diagnosis of ME/CFS should be reconsidered if none of the following key features are present:

- post-exertional fatigue or malaise,
- cognitive difficulties,
- sleep disturbance, and
- chronic pain [7].

4. International Consensus Criteria for ME/CFS:

This definition was also developed for both clinical and research purposes. To be diagnosed under the ICC definition, a patient will meet the criteria for post-exertional neuroimmune exhaustion (a), at least one symptom from three neurological impairment categories (b), at least one symptom from three immune/gastro-intestinal/genitourinary impairment categories (c), and at least one symptom from energy metabolism/transport impairments (d).

a) *post-exertional neuroimmune exhaustion (compulsory):*
This cardinal symptom features a pathological inability to produce, sufficient energy on demand with prominent symptoms primarily in the neuro-immune regions. Characteristics are:

i.   marked, rapid physical and/or cognitive fatiguability in response to exertion, which may be minimal such as activities of daily living or simple mental tasks, can be debilitating and cause relapse,
ii. post-exertional symptom exacerbation: e.g. acute flu-like symptoms, pain and worsening of other symptoms,
iii. post-exertional exhaustion may occur immediately after activity or be delayed by hours or days,

iv. recovery period is prolonged, usually taking 24 hours or longer. A relapse can last days, weeks or longer, and

v. low threshold of physical and mental fatigability (lack of stamina) results in a substantial reduction in pre-illness activity level.

b) *neurological impairments:*

At least one symptom from three of the following four symptom categories:

i. neurocognitive impairments: a) difficulty processing information: slowed thought, impaired concentration e.g. confusion, disorientation, cognitive overload, difficulty with making decisions, slowed speech, acquired or exertional dyslexia and b) short-term memory loss: e.g. difficulty remembering what one wanted to say, what one was saying, retrieving words, recalling information, poor working memory,

ii. pain: a) headaches: e.g. chronic, generalized headaches often involve aching of the eyes, behind the eyes or back of the head that may be associated with cervical muscle tension; migraine; tension headaches; and b) significant pain: can be experienced in muscles, muscle-tendon junctions, joints, abdomen or chest. It is non-inflammatory in nature and often migrates e. g. generalized hyperalgesia, widespread pain (may meet fibromyalgia criteria), myofascial or radiating pain,

iii. sleep disturbance: a) disturbed sleep patterns: e.g. insomnia, prolonged sleep including naps, sleeping most of the day and being awake most of the night, frequent awakenings, awakening much earlier than before illness onset, vivid dreams/nightmares and b) unrefreshing sleep: e.g. awaken feeling exhausted regardless of duration of sleep, day-time sleepiness, and

iv. neurosensory, perceptual and motor disturbances: a) neurosensory or perceptual: e.g. inability to focus vision, sensitivity to light, noise, vibration, odor, taste and touch; impaired depth perception and b) motor: e.g. muscle weakness, twitching, poor coordination, feeling unsteady on feet, ataxia.

c) *immune, gastro-intestinal and genitourinary impairments:*
At least one symptom from three of the following five symptom categories:

   i.   flu-like symptoms may be recurrent or chronic and typically, activate or worsen with exertion: e.g. sore throat, sinusitis, cervical and/or axillary lymph nodes may enlarge or be tender on palpitation

  ii.   susceptibility to viral infections with prolonged recovery periods

 iii.   gastro-intestinal tract: e.g. nausea, abdominal pain, bloating, irritable bowel syndrome

 iv.   genitourinary: e.g. urinary urgency or frequency, nocturia, and

  v.   sensitivities to food, medications, odors or chemicals.

d) *energy production/transportation impairments:*
At least one symptom from the following categories:

   i.   cardiovascular: e.g. inability to tolerate an upright position – orthostatic intolerance, neutrally-mediated hypotension, postural orthostatic tachycardia syndrome, palpitations with or without cardiac arrhythmias, light-headedness/dizziness,

  ii.   respiratory: e.g. air hunger, labored breathing, fatigue of chest wall muscles,

 iii.   loss of thermostatic ability: e.g. subnormal body temperature, marked diurnal fluctuations, sweating episodes, recurrent feelings of feverishness with or without low grade fever, cold extremities, and

 iv.   intolerance of temperature extremes [8, 9].

Sources:

1. Institute of Medicine of the National Academies: Committee on the diagnostic criteria for ME/CFS (2015). *Beyond ME/CFS: Redefining an illness.* Washington (DC): National Academies Press (US). February 2015.
2. Jason, L., M. Sunnquist, A. Brown, M. Evans, S. Vernon, J. Furst & V. Simonis (2013). Examining case definition criteria for CFS and ME. *Fatigue: Biomedicine, Health & Behavior,* 2(1).

3. Brurberg, K.G., M.S. Fonhus, L. Larun & S. Flottorp (2014). Case definitions for CFS/ME: A systemic review. B*MJ Open,* 4(2):1-12.

4. CDC (Centers for Disease Control and Prevention) (2012). Chronic fatigue syndrome: 1994 case definition. [December 16, 2013]. http://www.cdc.gov/cfs/case-definition/1994.html.

5. Fakuda, K., S. Straus, I. Hickie, M. Sharpe, J. Dobbins, L. Komaroff & the International Chronic Fatigue Syndrome Study Group (1994). The Chronic Fatigue Syndrome: A comprehensive approach to its definition and study. *Annals of Internal Medicine,* 121:953-959.

6. Jason, L., A, M. Evans, N. Porter, M. Brown, J. Hunnell, V. Anderson, A. Lerch, K. De Meirleir and F. Friedberg (2010). The development of a revised Canadian myalgic encephalomyelitis/chronic fatigue syndrome case definition. *American Journal of Biochemistry and Biotechnology,* 6:120–135.

7. https://me-pedia.org/wiki/NICE_guidelines. Note: The NICE guidelines are currently under review. The new guidelines are expected to be published in December 2020. (https://meassociation.org.uk/2019/12/new-nice-guidelines-on-me-cfs-delayed-until-end-2020-06-december-2019/).

8. Carruthers, B., M. van de Sande, K. De Meirleir, N. Klimas, G. Broderick, T. Mitchell, D. Staines, A. Powles, N. Speight, R. Vallings & L. Bateman (2011). Myalgic Encephalomyelitis: International Consensus Criteria. *Journal of Internal Medicine,* 284(4):327-338. doi: 10.1111/j.1365-2796.2011.02428. x. Article first published online: 20 July 2011.

9. Carruthers, B., M. van de Sande, K. De Meirleir, N. Klimas, G. Broderick, T. Mitchell, D. Staines, A. Powles, N. Speight, R. Vallings, L. Bateman, B. Baumgarten-Austrheim, D. Bell, N. Carlo-Stella, J. Chia, A. Darragh, D. Jo, D. Lewis, A. Light, S. Marshall-Gradisbik, I. Mena, J. Mikovits, K. Miwa, M. Murovska, M. Pall & S. Stevens (2017). Myalgic encephalomyelitis: International Consensus Criteria. *Journal of Internal Medicine,* 282(4):353. Article first published online: 20 September 2017. https://onlinelibrary.wiley.com/doi/ full/10.1111/joim.12658.

Made in the USA
Monee, IL
28 December 2020